SUNLIGHT AND HEALTH

By the Same Author

PARENTHOOD AND RACE-CULTURE
THE PROGRESS OF EUGENICS
THE EUGENIC PROSPECT

SUNLIGHT AND HEALTH

BY

C. W. SALEEBY
M.D., Ch.B., F.Z.S., F.R.S.E.

CHAIRMAN OF THE NATIONAL BIRTHRATE COMMISSION, 1918–20
CHAIRMAN OF THE SUNLIGHT LEAGUE.

WITH AN INTRODUCTION BY

THE LATE

SIR WILLIAM M. BAYLISS
M.A., D.Sc., F.R.S.

FORMERLY PROFESSOR OF GENERAL PHYSIOLOGY, UNIVERSITY COLLEGE,
LONDON, AND CHAIRMAN OF THE COMMITTEE ON LIGHT OF THE MEDICAL
RESEARCH COUNCIL OF GREAT BRITAIN.

THIRD EDITION

London
NISBET & CO. LTD
22, BERNERS STREET, W. 1.

First Published in - - 1923
Second Edition - - - 1924
Third ,, *December,* 1926

PRINTED IN GREAT BRITAIN BY THE WHITEFRIARS PRESS, LTD.,
LONDON AND TONBRIDGE.

To the Memory
OF
MY MOTHER,
A TRUE DOCTOR'S DAUGHTER,
WHO DENIED ME NO NATURAL
BOON IN CHILDHOOD

PREFACE TO THE THIRD EDITION

IN writing a preface to the third edition of this book it affords no small measure of satisfaction to record the notable advances made since the last edition was called for. We have lost, and yet we have not lost, the greatest of the long line of great physiologists produced by our country. Elsewhere [1] I have sought to pay due homage to the late Sir William Bayliss, in whom the Committee on Light of the Medical Research Council loses its first chairman and the voice to whose most potent support [2] was due the assent of the Council, early in 1922, to my plea for the initiation of the scientific study in this country of the relation of light to health. Had he lived, he would have been profoundly interested to learn from Dr. A. F. Hess, of Columbia University, whose laboratories he visited in 1922, that several American workers have succeeded in creating vitamins or their equivalents in foods destitute of them by means of exposure to light.

The systematic radiation of certain foods, and especially of winter milk, will be a commonplace in a few years. Various hospitals have begun it, and admirable results are recorded in the latest Report of the Medical Research Council. Artificial lamps

[1] *New Statesman.* "William Michael Bayliss," Sept. 13, 1924.
[2] See p. 80 of the text.

have a much wider sphere of utility than the clinical alone. At the English-Speaking Conference on Child Welfare, held in London last July, I urged that the installations of such lamps in our hospitals should be in practically continuous three-fold use : first, to treat patients ; second, to compensate night nurses, in especial, for their lack of sunlight ; and third, for the radiation of the food supplied to the patients and staff. Already, as a matter of course, the winter milk for young and old in my own home is radiated by a mercury vapour quartz lamp.

But the sun is best. Admirable results are recorded from the Zoological Gardens, following the use of the vitaglass which I asked our chemists, in 1924 (see p. xviii), to construct. I have been visiting the Gardens for more than forty years and the animals have never been so healthy, happy and beautiful as now. The admission to mammals, birds and reptiles alike, even of the exiguous supply of ultra-violet light that reaches Regent's Park under the present barbaric conditions of coal-combustion, has been triumphantly successful.[1] Dr. J. Ferguson, School Medical Officer for Smethwick, reports excellent results also from his schools. The Development Commissioners are officially suggesting the use of ultra-violet rays for our cows in the winter. First, we should use vitaglass for cowsheds, obviously. Then we can reiterate and amplify the question which I have been asking ever since the glass

---

[1] The glass was invented by Mr. F. E. Lamplough, M.A., formerly Fellow of Trinity College, Cambridge, and is obtainable from Messrs. Chance, Smethwick, Birmingham.

of life proved so successful at the Zoological Gardens
—If for chimpanzees and cows, why not for children ?
Are they not worth " a wilderness of monkeys " ?

But nothing avails unless the ultra-violet light is
really allowed to reach us from the sky. These
notes for the third edition of this little book are
being prepared after the Bill has passed through Committee in the House of Commons a Smoke Abatement
Bill, introduced by the Minister of Health, Mr. Neville
Chamberlain. It is much overdue, fifty-one years
after the futile clauses of the Public Health Act of
1875, and thirty-six years after the great discovery
of Dr. Palm. My view of the measure may be
gathered from the correspondence which has passed
between Mr. Chamberlain and myself on behalf of
the Sunlight League, and which was published in *The
Times*, October 30th, 1926. The Bill will do good in
respect of the industrial chimney. It promises to
be impotent—in respect of the graver offender, the
domestic chimney. (See *Sunlight*, No. 3.)

Mr. Chamberlain has been inadequately informed
by his advisers. When he introduced the Bill in the
House of Commons, he said that we lose, in our
cities, 20 per cent. of the sunlight enjoyed by the
countryside. This figure refers merely to the
calorific power of the sun, which is irrelevant.
So much for Dr. Palm's demand in 1890 ! But when
that demand is complied with, as under the auspices
of the Committee on Light, it is found that we lose
in our cities not 20 per cent., but something of the
order of 80 per cent. of the vital rays which fall upon
the countryside.

The abolition of urban smoke is, therefore, in this most fundamental respect, four times as important as Mr. Chamberlain himself suggests. An official record and analysis of the really relevant readings of the past two years is now in the Press. Would that it might appear in time to strengthen the hands of the Minister of Health against the vested interests of the powers of darkness, now in league against him and us and our children after us !

As ever, public opinion must be educated and organised. For further progress I place my hopes in a specially created instrument, of which the record must now be made.

Thirty-six years ago Dr. Theobald Adrian Palm, in the memorable paper (*The Practitioner*, October and November, 1890) in which he showed that rickets is due to deprivation of sunlight, stated the objects at which, in my view, a League in support of sunlight treatment should aim.

On May 14th, 1924, the Sunlight League was formed at Carnegie House, Piccadilly,[1] on a resolution proposed by myself.

In abbreviated form the following (as the reader will see hereafter) were Dr. Palm's proposals :—

The recording of sunshine in the streets and alleys of smoky cities, as well as at health resorts ; using means to indicate the chemical activity of the sun's rays rather than its heat.[2]

[1] Late Patron: H.M. Queen Alexandra; Presidents: The Duke of Sutherland and Dr. T. A. Palm; Chairman: C. W. Saleeby, M.D., F.R.S.E.; Offices: 29 Gordon Square, W.C.1.; Journal *Sunlight*.
[2] This has now been begun at the National Institute for Medical

The removal of rickety children from large towns to Sanatoria in sunlit places.

The systematic use of sunbaths as a preventive and therapeutic measure in rickets and other diseases.

The education of the public to the appreciation of sunlight as a means of health ; teaching the nation that sunlight is Nature's universal disinfectant, as well as a stimulant and tonic.

Such knowledge will also stimulate efforts for the abatement of smoke and for the multiplication of open spaces, especially as playgrounds for the children of the poor.

To these great proposals, made a generation ago, I could contribute nothing but a few obvious addenda : smoke and slums must go ; sunlight is our common need and heritage ; the League's objects are national, above party, class or creed ; open spaces in great cities must be used as never before ; so long as we continue to breed the diseases of darkness, sanatoria and hospitals must be set up in the sunniest parts of the country, which is now being surveyed for that purpose ; children specially must be treated outside our smoky cities (smoke-cursed Sheffield, of which some hard words are written in the early pages of this book, is proposing to transfer all its four hospitals, beginning with the Children's, to a park outside the city) ; the " dark Satanic mills," especially in the North, must be transformed, as has been done in other countries ; we must establish schools in the sun ; the nation's new houses should be so placed as to receive

Research, Hampstead, and the readings are published in *The Times* every morning.

the sun and so equipped as not to eclipse it by smoke ;
the clothing especially of children must be studied
afresh ; we must support the principles of daylight
saving and the cultivation of allotments ; we must
seek a cheap substitute for window-glass, such that it
may be transparent to ultra-violet rays [1] ; we must
steadily strive to protect and supply those many who
cannot go to the Mediterranean every winter ; and
must urge the claims of the light of life upon Parliament, the Press, and health and housing Committees
throughout the country, until it may be said again,
as of old, " The people that walked in darkness have
seen a great light, and they that dwell in the land of
the shadow of death, upon them hath the light
shined."

One week after its foundation the Sunlight League
held its first meeting, and it was then my privilege as
chairman publicly to introduce Dr. Palm, who still,
in his seventy-ninth year, visits his patients on his
bicycle around Aylesford, in Kent, the " Garden of
England "—and Dr. Rollier, the first Vice-President
of the League. Little more than five years have
passed since, having visited Leysin, I began to
publish in the *Observer*, *New Statesman*, *Outlook*,
Daily News, *Manchester Guardian*, *Daily Chronicle*,
Medical Press, and elsewhere, a series of articles
describing and commending his work. His name was
then entirely unknown in this country to the public,
and to all but perhaps half a dozen members of the
medical profession. Immense volumes were published about tuberculosis, in which sunlight was

[1] See my letter in *Nature*, May, 24th 1924.

never mentioned. Air, food, water, and so forth, were discussed in respect of health ; sunlight was never mentioned. Any one who questions this fact, which now seems so surprising, need only look at the official and non-official literature on health, and notably on tuberculosis and on childhood, published in this country until 1922. In the autumn of 1921 Dr. Rollier was first named in *The Times* in a letter in which I called his " La Cure de Soleil " the most valuable book on tuberculosis ever published— which, of course, it is, and without any important second. Let us remember that the bacteriologists have been offering us their preparations from Koch himself in 1890 to Dr. Georges Dreyer in 1923, and the less said of most of them the better.

It was in 1890, also, that Dr. Palm published his paper on sunlight and rickets. He had observed the absence of rickets during his nine years (from about 1875) as a medical missionary in Japan, and had contrasted that fact with the dreadful frequency of the disease in the slums of Edinburgh, where he had studied. It still abounds in the Cowgate, as in his time there, and in mine. When I exhumed his memorable paper from the files of the *Practitioner*, where it had lain buried for a generation, I found it still alive and luminous. The geographical method, used by a country doctor in Cumberland, after his return from Japan, had anticipated all the German and American laboratories by decades. Britain bears the Palm.

The contentions of the following pages are under-statements. Many critics protest against exaggeration ; they have not been to Leysin. They have not read the remarkable paper [1] in which it is shown by Dr. Leonard Hill and his colleagues that even one dose of light will markedly raise the bactericidal power of the blood. The hypothesis that light acts by injuring the skin, and inducing a kind of vaccination-reaction by absorption of toxins from the cutaneous damage, as other counter-irritants act, thus defining the sun and sky of Leysin as a celestial sinapism, seems to me, however, with all respect, to be an instance of obsession by certain nineteenth century ideas. We shall be told next that our food acts by poisoning us, and our drinking water by drowning us. But the observed experimental facts are very valuable.

Everywhere now hospitals are installing light clinics, usually in an abandoned cellar, coal-hole or the like. At the Infant's Hospital, Westminster, where I lectured on this subject in 1923, the Medical Director, Dr. Eric Pritchard, puts out on the iron fire-escape infants whom the superb equipment of that hospital cannot cure in its wards ; practitioners are buying a vast variety of lamps as fast as they can and using them, in many instances, with little reference to the temperature factor. The results promise to be very various. Many practitioners are suggesting that artificial phototherapy is preferable to the use of sunlight ; they belong by instinct and education to the same group as those who prefer arti-

[1] "The Effect of Radiation on the Bactericidal Power of the Blood," by L. Colebrook, A. Eidinow, and Leonard Hill (*British Journal of Experimental Pathology*, 1924, Vol. V., p. 54).

ficial feeding of the infant to breast-feeding; and they use similar arguments. Let us get back to the Sun.

Sunlight is our common heritage and our common need. The nation's children, our future all, need it even more than the fortunate few who can repair to their villas on the Riviera when the " November particulars " return. The Sunlight League has been formed to point to the light of day, not so much to advocate heliotherapy as what I have called heliohygiene—the use of sunlight for preventive medicine and constructive health, the building of whole and happy bodies from the cradle and before it. The League is aimed against no interests but such as rob us of our sunlight, turn our cities in winter into cold hells and call the process industry, or imprison children in shadow and call the process education. During the summer of 1924 the League gave the sunlight of Kenwood to a few dozen children by way of demonstrating what millions of children should receive next year and ever after. I ask my readers to support this campaign for sunlight and for education about it. We must remind ourselves, yet again, in our zeal for the light of the sun and our hatred of the diseases of darkness, that Shakespeare said, " There is no darkness but ignorance." For myself, I wish not to fill Dr. Rollier's cliniques—as seemed to be happening when I paid my last visit to them in August of this year—but to empty them, and to see him receive the Nobel Prize by way of consolation.

C. W. S.

ROYAL INSTITUTION, LONDON, W.
December, 1926.

PREFACE TO THE FIRST EDITION

BEFORE finally passing the proofs of this little book, which seeks to serve so great an advance in medicine and hygiene by means of an idea at once simple and profound, yet new—Pardon, O shades of Akhenaton and Zoroaster and Hippocrates !—I have thought it well to spend a week in Copenhagen, in order to see for myself the present work at the Finsen Medical Light Institute. My thanks are due, for many hours of interest and instruction, in the clinical department of dermatology to Dr. Axel Reyn, Director of the Institute, in the surgical clinic to Dr. Chievitz, and in the research laboratory to Dr. Carl Sonne, to whose remarkable work I have been drawing attention for some years, and to Dr. Poul Schultzer, his assistant.

My observations under the guidance of these followers of Finsen have most amply confirmed the views expressed in the following pages. In an Appendix references are given to the most recent work in this magnificent institution, confirming and extending the earlier work of Dr. Sonne himself, and of Dr. Hess and his colleagues in New York. It may be particularly insisted that the visible light rays seem to have very special qualities against infectious disease, such as tuberculosis, which must not be forgotten because we can so clearly show the specific value of the ultra-violet rays in respect of the chemistry of the blood and the prevention and cure of rickets. If we collate the work of Sonne with that of the Americans and others, we see that, doubtless, the *whole* of the solar radiation, as it reaches us after filtration through a natural smokeless atmosphere, is valuable for our lives—as might well be expected on general evolutionary principles. As the Greeks concluded that *ariston men hudor*—water is best, so we may conclude, after study of various artificially produced portions of the solar radiation, that *aristos men helios*—the sun is best.

My comparative observation of the patients in the surgical wards at the Finsen Institute, where the general light bath is used, by means of the carbon arc lamp, and of the much more fortunate patients at Leysin, where the sun himself shines and heals, convinces me afresh that indeed the sun is best, and that the most useful purpose of the artificial lamps, of whatever kind, is to guide our footsteps back to the light of day.

One correction to something implied in the text should be made. Certain papers [1] by Finsen have been put before me which show that he did not only regard the sunlight—or artificial light—as an antiseptic, but also recognised its power as "incitement"—arousing the power of resistance to disease. That is the truth which most of us have forgotten, though the power of the general light bath, as distinguished from mere local "antiseptic" treatment, has been

[1] See, for instance, his "Lyset som Incitament," *Hospitalstidende*, No. 8, 1895, Copenhagen.

employed, through the sun, by Rollier since 1903, and at the Finsen Institute since 1913.

A recent visit to Finland, famous, *inter alia*, for its athletic prowess and splendid vital statistics, despite its cold winters, confirms the teaching of Chapter VIII., derived from Canada, for the winters of Finland are sunny.

To many clinicians and researchers in many lands, Denmark, Switzerland, and the United States in especial, whose clinics and laboratories have been at my disposal for comparative observation ; to Sir William Bayliss, Sir James Crichton-Browne, and Sir Arthur Keith for much encouragement and help in my own country ; to very many editors who have published my arguments, during the past four years in especial, in various forms ; and to those organisations who have invited me to their platforms for the purpose of public education in this regard, my thanks are most sincerely now conveyed. No book could be adequate for the demonstration of the value of sunlight, which properly teaches its worth through its own special child, the eye, looking upon its visible results ; and certainly my book is not. But with all its imperfections, at least it points aright to the light of life.

C. W. S.

COPENHAGEN,
September, 1923.

P.S.—As " Lens," it has been my special pleasure to write on this subject elsewhere—a fact noted here in order to relieve my not unnatural jealousy of that writer.

CONTENTS

INTRODUCTION

THE author of this book is well known for his persistent and powerful advocacy of the great importance of sunlight for health. He may well be congratulated on the abundant justification of his action afforded by the discoveries of the last few years, and on the general recognition now given to his main contentions. The book aims at giving a brief account of the interesting field of phenomena as a whole. I am unaware of the existence of any similar work with so wide a scope, and it should be of much use to those desirous of obtaining a genearl view.

It will be seen that while the most striking effects of light have shown themselves in the actual cure of diseased conditions, such as rickets and tuberculosis, it is known that light prevents the development of these in circumstances in which they would otherwise assuredly show themselves. It seems clear, therefore, that we must ascribe to sunlight very important functions in the preservation of normal health.

Hence, we see the justification for the efforts being made to prevent atmospheric pollution by smoke—efforts in which Dr. Saleeby has taken a prominent part.

All readers will, as it seems to me, notice that, however certain we are of the facts themselves, there is a great deal yet to be learned as to the way in which light acts, and as to the particular rays of the spectrum which are active in different cases. It is to be hoped that Dr. Saleeby's book will serve a further valuable purpose in directing attention to the gaps in our knowledge, and in exciting research to fill them up.

W. M. BAYLISS.

"In the beginning, God said, Let there be light."—
The Book of Genesis

"Our toil from thought all glorious forms shall cull
To make this Earth, our Home, more beautiful,
And Science and her sister Poesy
Shall clothe in light the fields and cities of the free."
SHELLEY: *The Revolt of Islam*

SUNLIGHT AND HEALTH

CHAPTER I

INTRODUCTORY

IN this volume, designed for the medical profession and the public, to commend sunlight as the primary and hitherto most neglected means of health and medicine against disease, the attempt is made, with the most recent data, to state the case for a lifelong conviction of the author, which he has steadily followed in his own domestic ways. No new discovery does he here attribute to himself. No argument about priority seems appropriate to any modern when we learn that Hippocrates, the Father of Medicine, used the sunlight. The only personal claim here made is that the subject has hitherto been neglected, to our immense loss, that a few clinicians here and there have used sunlight, that none of them have understood its action, that only by exact scientific research can its action be understood, and that persistent reiteration on the part of an observer who, having learnt much, asked for more, has given us an authoritative scientific committee, under the ægis of the Privy Council of the United Kingdom of Great Britain and Ireland, to study the subject, and to find the scientific bases

upon which, it is here predicted, a much vaster and
more valuable edifice than even heliotherapy, as we
know it to-day, may be erected. Our knowledge of
the subject is at present merely fragmentary and
rudimentary. Many positive and dogmatic asser-
tions are made in the following pages ; much action,
some of it revolutionary to our current ideas, is
demanded ; but the main purpose, here explicitly
asserted, is to ask for " MORE LIGHT," even more in
the metaphorical than in the literal sense of the
dying Goethe's famous phrase.

As a medical student in Edinburgh—"Auld
Reekie," or "Old Smoky," as the natives of the
modern Athens call it with somewhat fatuous
affection—I always abominated the smoke which,
inter alia, distinguishes the Calton Hill from the
Acropolis and its unfinished columns from the
Parthenon. In 1898, during one of the wet Saturday
afternoons which make cricket so difficult an exotic
in Scotland, I saw a typical smoke-stained urban
lung in the Pathological Museum of the University,
and resolved never to buy an ounce of coal for my
own use—a resolution steadily kept until this day.
During those student years in Edinburgh I learnt to
hate tuberculosis, the " glands in the neck," " white
swelling " of the knee-joint, psoas abscesses, and so
forth, that ever crowded out the wards and the
out-patient departments ; at the Royal Maternity
Hospital, in 1901, the tragic end of the first case in
the first ante-natal bed in the world made me hate
rickets [1] ; and during a term as resident physician

---

[1] See p. 6.

at the Royal Infirmary in the following year, when I was allowed to put patients on the balconies in all weathers, and when one tuberculous child of five, terribly wasted and with an immense abdomen, recovered on the end balcony of Ward 16, without surgery, but with air and light and cod-liver oil, my natural instinct for the open air and for following Nature in the search for Life, her daughter, was powerfully fortified.

Leaving for London, also in 1901, almost the first place I visited was the Finsen Ward of the London Hospital, where light was to be seen curing lupus, a form of cutaneous tuberculosis. In the *World's Work* I then sought to draw public attention to the meaning of this work ; and again, when Finsen died in 1904, I drew attention to the possibility that the light which he used acted not only as an antiseptic against the bacilli but as a stimulant to the patient's tissues. Numerous occasional articles and lectures in succeeding years relieved my mind, perhaps, but did no more. No legislation was effected, in respect of either the domestic or the industrial chimney ; no treatment by light beyond the artificial phototherapy of lupus was used in this country. A pretentious new façade was built to St. Mary's Hospital, in London, to commemorate a royal personage, on exactly the same principle as that which Florence Nightingale had condemned for Netley Hospital half a century earlier. Everybody advocated fresh air, some advocated open air, Professor Leonard Hill greatly advanced our understanding of the value of moving air, but neither he nor any one else used or studied sunlight in this country.

Paying a first visit to New York in 1919, I was first astonished at the rule under which the train that took me thither from Halifax had to wait, many miles outside the city, whilst electric locomotion was substituted for the coal-smoke-producing engine, the nearer approach of which was forbidden by the sanitary regulations of the metropolis. Less than an hour later I was again astonished at the smokeless, sunlit cleanliness of the great city, by way of contrast to London, that "suburb of Hell," as John Evelyn called it centuries ago. Leaving the city for home and seeing the sun set clear behind the astonishingly clear façade of its skyscrapers, I remembered that we were to build new houses in England, and that here was a possible part-answer to the devastating old argument which had faced me so often in so many years—that we could not afford to reconstruct our old houses so as to make them smokeless in habitation. At least we could start aright with our new ones. Since that voyage I have devoted nearly all my time to a continuous inquiry into the relations of sunlight to health and disease, and continued public demand for action, curative and preventive, according to the results of such inquiry. In 1921, in my volume "The Eugenic Prospect," [1] I stated the case as forcibly and completely as I then could, and there is no need to go over that ground again.

[1] London, Fisher Unwin & Co. ; New York, Dodd, Mead & Co. See Part II., "Let There Be Light."

Eugenics was my first love, for whom I forsook the practice of medicine, having yet scarcely begun it. The late Sir Francis Galton's lecture to the Sociological Society, in 1904, inaugurating modern eugenics, settled that question for me. Twenty years after, we are no nearer the original Galtonian eugenics—positive eugenics, as I called it with his consent.[1] He was right when, in another communication, soon after the first, he told us that, for success, the eugenic idea must affect us with the force of a religion. Without some such effective emotional stimulus we may discuss and study eugenics, but we do not practise it. I see not the remotest prospect, in any land, of any such effective sentiment as Galton saw the need for, if eugenics was to deserve the name of action. But, failing positive eugenics, the encouragement of worthy parenthood, as I have defined it, there remain certain possibilities which, for what they are worth, we must pursue. There is negative eugenics, the discouragement of unworthy parenthood, as by the permanent segregation of the feeble-minded. There is the study of the development of childhood and youth, so that at least parenthood may later be possible without preventable risk or defect. Here we touch upon the relations of sunlight to the normal processes of development. We must, for instance, study the effect of sunlight upon the ductless glands, which have potent controlling and directive relations

[1] See " Parenthood and Race Culture : An Outline of Eugenics," 1909 (Cassell, London ; Moffatt, Yard, New York), the first book on eugenics, dedicated to Galton, who read it before publication. (Out of print.)

to the reproductive system. Also we must recognise the significance of rickets in relation to parenthood. When I was resident physician in the Royal Maternity Hospital, Edinburgh, in 1901, there was inaugurated the first bed, in any hospital in the world, devoted to the expectant mother. That ante-natal bed has now grown into a ward, and is copied all the world over. The pioneer to whom it was solely due was Dr. John William Ballantyne, first of modern men to recognise the truth, well known to Moses, that life begins in the womb, and our care of it must begin there too. As a matter of history, let me here record that the first patient to occupy that first ante-natal bed in the world was a little rickety woman from smoky Leeds. Failing any other possibility of deliverance, Cæsarean section was performed. She died, and soon afterwards her hapless infant died in my arms. Such was the inauspicious beginning of a great epoch in the care of motherhood. But rickets is a disease of darkness. An Edinburgh graduate had taught the truth about it in 1890, and been ignored in Edinburgh and everywhere else. The restoration of sunlight to its primary place in hygiene and medicine must mean the end of rickets, and thus the end of all those cases where rickety contraction and distortion of the female pelvis involves the gravest risks to motherhood and the maintenance of the race.

In 1921 I first saw Leysin, directed thereto by Dr. Ceresole, of Lausanne, with whom I had discussed my campaign for what I call helio-hygiene, based upon such considerations as the notable acceleration in the decline of tuberculosis in New York, which, during visits and inquiries in that city in the two previous years, I had found to follow the sanitary regulation of 1905 forbidding the production of coal-smoke. Nowhere on earth have I seen, nor heard tell, of anything so beautiful, so significant, so hopeful, as the application of heliotherapy under the charge of Dr. Rollier. On the following day I first opened his book, "La Cure de Soleil," published shortly before the war, and submerged in that destructive deluge. Only a few minutes were needed to breed the determination that the book which taught what my eyes had just seen in the flesh—the whole, healed, happy flesh of hundreds—at Leysin, must appear in English, for the needs of all who speak that tongue on both sides of the Atlantic, and especially for us in the British Isles, whose cities, thanks to our self-imposed curse of coal-smoke, and to our infamous slums, are the darkest on earth. The publication, in 1923, of Rollier's " Heliotherapy " is the satisfaction—and more, for it is really a new book—of that desire. Meanwhile, it has been my privilege to see the work of other heliotherapeutists and to realise, more certainly than ever, the significance of such practice as theirs for the life of man whenever and wherever he builds and inhabits cities—as he must, for what does the very word civilisation mean ? From these lessons he " must learn or perish."

The superb results of Sir Henry Gauvain at Alton and Hayling Island showed me that *vastly* much more extensive, systematic and fundamental inquiry into the scientific foundations of the sun-cure was necessary—for evidently even our English sun, and even at sea level, can heal. After a few months' re-iteration, a demand for the proper organisation of such an inquiry was met by the Medical Research Council, which appointed, early in 1922, a Committee on Sunlight, with Sir William Bayliss as its chairman. Vastly more than even the unequalled relief and cure of surgical tuberculosis is involved in this question, but only when the scientific foundations are laid can we build the structure of heliotherapy and, better still, of helio-hygiene, which will afford for us the full gamut of the value of sunlight, and make an end of the diseases of darkness—" *les maladies de l'ombre*," as Dr. Rollier translates my phrase—from tuberculosis, the prince of the powers of dark-ness, down to rickets, the widespread curse and ugly scandal of our British malurbanisation.

The promise of this subject cannot fail to interest and stimulate the many and energetic men who are rapidly making English-speaking North America the leader and tutor of all the world. Shortly before my first visit to Leysin I had learnt, in Winnipeg, how indignantly the health authorities of that splendid young city were dealing with a very trifling and transient pollution of the air, and obstruction of sunlight by coal-smoke. Since that date I have learnt, in Boston, how the " Floating Hospital " (a ship at anchor in its historic harbour) serves to expose ailing children to the sunlight, which is guaranteed to them by the city's " Blue Sky Law," and to cure them by its incomparable means. And as recently as December, 1922, I had the advantage of seeing the work of Dr. Alfred F. Hess, of New York, and of his colleagues, in Columbia University, and at the Home for Hebrew Infants, where he has shown that the quantity of phosphorus in the blood of babies *rises* from winter to summer and *falls* from summer to winter, whilst the incidence of rickets (" *la maladie de l'ombre par excellence,*" as Dr. Rollier has described it to me) consentaneously falls and rises. (It was an Englishman, Dr. Theobald Adrian Palm, who, in 1890, in the *Practitioner, a generation ago*, first taught the relation of rickets to darkness and to sunlight ; but no one heeded him.)

The very few who have protested in England that we were sinning against the light, are now seen to be right : John Evelyn, who wrote his " Fumifugium " in 1661, and condemned the " hellish cloud of sea-coal that maketh the City of London resemble the suburbs of hell " ; and John Ruskin, who inveighed against the " plague clouds " that ascended from our industrial cities, and was thought to be a fool for his pains ; and Sir Benjamin Ward Richardson, one of the few doctors who have had Latin enough to know that doctor means teacher ; and Sir William Blake Richmond, the painter who knew that, as St. Augustine said, " Light is the queen of colours." Dr. Rollier and his followers have vindicated them all ; and in praise of the sunlight the half has not yet been said. Who could have guessed, a year or two ago, that a few minutes' exposure to it daily will double the quantity of

phosphorus in a baby's blood in a fortnight ; or cure
rickets as rapidly and certainly and costlessly as Dr.
Harriette Chick and her fellow-workers, sent from
London to help and to learn from the hapless children
of Vienna, have lately demonstrated ?

Our houses, our hospitals—consider the wards of
St. George's Hospital at Hyde Park Corner, and
contrast them, in the light of the following pages,
with Hyde Park itself, unused for cure—our schools,
our factories, our clothes, all these and more must
be reconsidered as we emerge from the last—for
surely it must be the last—of the Dark Ages into
the light of day. For evidently the real meaning of
Dr. Rollier's work is not clinical but hygienic ; I
praise it, here and everywhere, in order to end it,
leaving him nothing to do but to write his memoirs.

Meanwhile it is a serious question whether, in
Britain, so long as we continue to make many of
our children tuberculous, we should not send them
to Switzerland, where they can be cured by the sun
in a year or two, rather than treat them for many
years until they die in any of the various dark
places on which we rely at present, and some of
which it has been my miserable experience recently
to visit in search of more light. That question must
be reiterated, at whatever cost of offence to vested
and other interests. One kind of difficulty which
the champions of the light in Britain must over-
come may be illustrated by a single sentence from
Dr. F. E. Wynne, Medical Officer of Health and
Professor of Public Health in Sheffield, that smoke-
cursed, rickets-and-tuberculosis-haunted survival of

nineteenth century industrialism and waste at their worst :

No one who has the true interests of our tuberculous population at heart can fail to regret Dr. Saleeby's suggestion that sunshine can cure tuberculosis. (*Manchester Guardian*, April 24th, 1922.)

What can be said of the fact that a high authority could write such words nineteen years after Dr. Rollier began curing tuberculosis by sunlight, not more than twenty-four hours away from our shores ? Or what can be said of those who persist in confounding light and heat (as if Shakespeare had written "Fear no more the *light* of the sun"), unable to learn from, for instance, the natural practice of the animals in our Zoological Gardens, who seek the early morning light of the sun but avoid its midday heat ? Or of those who persist in confounding light and air, like the critic of my lecture on sunlight at the Congress of the Royal Sanitary Institute in 1922, who declined to perceive anything new to learn, for she had herself "been preaching fresh air for thirty-five years" ? Or of those who, never having seen heliotherapy in practice, nor having read a line by any of its students, begin by exposing the chests of phthisical patients to the midday sun for an hour or so, and then infer from the subsequent pyrexia, hæmoptysis and autopsy that sunlight is useless in pulmonary tuberculosis ? Or of those who proclaim satisfaction with the ghastly records of our sanatorium system in this country, unaware that every sanatorium which is not in essence a solarium must to-day be called a tragic farce ? Or of the authorities at a large sanatorium for tuberculous children, mercilessly set on our bleak north-eastern coast, whither I was driven fourteen miles from a great northern port explicitly in order to see the sun-cure, and was told by the teacher in the school which is part of the institution that, when the sun shone, the children were sent into a neighbouring wood, by the doctors' orders, lest the light should hurt their eyes ?

No comment seems adequate but Schiller's, " Mit der Dummheit kämpfen Götter selbst vergebens."

I adhere to my oft-reiterated *dictum* in reference to Britain (contrasting, for instance, smoky London with smokeless New York, and smoky Sheffield with smokeless Essen), that the restoration of sunlight to our malurbanised millions, now blackened, bleached and blighted in slums and smoke, is the next great task of hygiene in our country.

CHAPTER II

SUNLIGHT AND DISEASE [1]

"IN the beginning, God said, Let There Be Light." In or before the eighth century B.C., Zarathustra, foremost among many sun-worshippers in many ages, taught the cult of the sun and the green leaf and thrift, in place of pillage and murder. In the beginning of medicine, Hippocrates, practising at Cos in the temple of Æsculapius—son of Phœbus Apollo, god of the sun and medicine and music—practised the sun-cure. In the beginning of our era, Galen and Celsus used the sun. In the Dark Ages, by a pitiful misconception, the cult of the sun fell into desuetude as a species of pagan Nature-worship, and ill persons were treated alike in physical and in intellectual night. Tuberculosis and other ills were treated by the sovereign touch, reputed to cure the "king's evil."

[1] This chapter, a general statement of the theme to be more particularly treated hereafter, is based upon the Friday Evening Discourse at the Royal Institution of Great Britain and Ireland, March 9th, 1923, Sir Arthur Keith, F.R.S., presiding. See also the *Proceedings of the Royal Institution*, 1923, and *Nature*, April 28th, 1923. The title of the Discourse was that preferred by the late Sir James Dewar, Fullerian Professor of Chemistry at the Royal Institution, to whom I owe much valuable help on the chemical aspects of the question. He wished the title of the Discourse to be in line with Tyndall's " Dust and Disease," of a much earlier date. A few days after the delivery of my Discourse Sir James Dewar died. To his memory I pay tribute here.

In the second half of the nineteenth century, we find certain heralds of the dawn. In 1856, Florence Nightingale vigorously but vainly protested against the orientation of Netley Hospital, observing that no sunlight could ever enter its wards. In 1876, Sir Benjamin Ward Richardson praised sunlight in his " Hygeia, the City of Health." In 1877, Downes and Blunt showed that sunlight will kill anthrax bacilli. In many writings at this period, John Ruskin upheld sunlight and declaimed against the " plague-cloud " of smoke above our cities. In 1890, Dr. Theobald Adrian Palm (*nat.* 1848), who still practises medicine at Aylesford, in the Garden of England, showed by the geographical method that lack of sunlight is the chief factor in the causation of rickets, and added an admirable series of recommendations accordingly.[1] His paper was entirely ignored, and I found it in America, thanks to an American bibliographer. Robert Koch and others showed that sunlight kills tubercle bacilli. In 1893, Niels Finsen began to cure lupus, a form of cutaneous tuberculosis, by the local use of sunlight, and Sir James Crichton-Browne made observations to the same effect in this country. In 1900, on May 1st, the London Hospital began the cure of lupus by the local use of sunlight, thanks to the really effective sovereign touch of Queen Alexandra, who was instrumental in bringing her young fellow-countryman's idea from Copenhagen.

In 1903, Dr. A. Rollier opened at Leysin, in the

[1] " The Geographical Distribution and Ætiology of Rickets," *The Practitioner*, October and November, 1890.

Alpes Vaudoises, the first clinic for the treatment of so-called surgical tuberculosis by sunlight ; and in 1910 he applied his idea to prevention by the establishment of the " school in the sun," at Cergnat, just below Leysin. In 1914, he published his book, " La Cure de Soleil," but the world catastrophe of that year caused it to be overlooked. In this country his methods have been followed recently by Sir Henry Gauvain, at the Treloar Hospital at Alton and Hayling Island, where very simple sheds and solaria serve to achieve results never approached by Netley, the pretentious and misplaced architecture of which exists in the same county to point the contrast between its century—the last of the ages of darkness—and the dawn in our own. In a very few other places, also, such as the Queen Mary's Hospital for Children at Carshalton, under Dr. Gordon Pugh—photographs of which from the air show a series of three-sided solaria strongly resembling the health temple at Cos,—at Leasowe, near Liverpool, at Perrysburg, near Buffalo, in the United States, and, following a recent lecture of mine, at the Heritage Craft Schools, Chailey, Sussex, the sun-cure is employed. At several others, which I have visited, the sun-cure is said to be employed, but is not, the elements of the matter being unknown to the persons in charge.

The results of heliotherapy, as seen by myself, or recorded in Rollier's radiographic and clinical atlas of 1914, or shown by means of illustrations, are unapproached, for certainty, safety, ease, beauty, restoration of function, and happiness during and after treatment. No explanation of them, to be called intelligible or adequate, is offered by any of its practitioners. Being myself without patients or laboratories, I have used only the geographical method, and have found, at each place studied, a tendency to believe that the various factors there present are essential for the results obtained. In the mountains, altitude is insisted upon ; at the sea, the argument for " helio-Alpine " is replaced by an argument for " helio-Marine." In high latitudes, the Mediterranean is described as impossible for sun-cure ; on visiting the Mediterranean, I found the sun-cure gloriously successful on the French and Italian Riviera, and there are similar reports from Spain. The fundamental bases were lacking for a superlatively successful empirical practice, conducted by various clinicians under widely varying conditions and in ignorance, for the most part, of each other's methods. No rational statement of the scope of heliotherapy could be obtained, some strongly denying, while Rollier strongly averred, that tuberculosis is amenable to the treatment when it happens to be situated in the lungs, as it is amenable when situated elsewhere. In his volume of 1914, Rollier mentioned certain other conditions besides tuberculosis, such as rickets, a non-bacterial disease, but the only explanation of the sun-cure that he offered was based on the antiseptic action of sunlight, while Gauvain explicitly regarded the sunlight as only of secondary value in his method.

Clearly the need was for a properly co-ordinated scientific inquiry into the action of sunlight upon the body in health and disease. We were using it as we used digitalis for the heart before pharmacology (to compare a great thing with one relatively trivial); we needed a true physio-pharmacology of this incomparable medicament. My demands (*e.g.*, in *Nature*, December 8th, 1921, p. 466; January 5th, 1922, p. 11) for such an inquiry were met, after six months, by the Medical Research Council, early in 1922, and from the date of the appointment of the Special Committee, under the chairmanship of Sir William Bayliss, a new chapter in clinical and preventive medicine, I believe, will be seen to begin, its provisional opening being the new and largely rewritten translation into English of " La Cure de Soleil," [1] on which I resolved immediately after my first visit to Leysin.

Already we have at least made it clear to all critics that the action is due to the sun's light and not to its heat. So long ago as 1779, Ingenhouss showed, as I am reminded by Sir James Dewar, that the dissociation of carbon dioxide by the green leaf is due to the sun's light and not to its heat. Yet, in several instances, the sun-cure has been tried, with calamitous results, by clinicians who, making no inquiry into the matter, have exposed the unaccustomed chests of phthisical patients to the midday sun, perhaps for an hour or two, with natural results in fever and hæmoptysis. Already, also, the idea that the light is less valuable in killing the infective agent than in raising the bodily resistance to it—an

---

[1] " Heliotherapy," by Dr. A. Rollier, with forewords by Sir H. J. Gauvain and Dr. C. W. Saleeby. Oxford Medical Publications, 1923.

idea to which I invited attention nearly twenty years ago, at the death of Finsen—has come into the clinical mind. Since August, 1922, in the Light Department of the London Hospital—which has done such splendid though limited work on the older hypothesis, since 1900—the general light bath has been used as well as the local treatment, and cases which resisted the latter have been completely cured by general exposure of the nude skin to the electric arc lamp, without local irradiation. We must use a combination of light and cold, which I have been commending for some time on the evidence of visits to Canada, where a magnificent childhood, free from rickets, thrives in extreme cold, thanks, as I believe, to a brilliant sun.

In various American laboratories the subject is now being advanced : notably in Columbia University, New York, under Dr. Alfred F. Hess and his fellow-workers.[1] They attribute the major part of the action of the sun to the ultra-violet rays, by which, in experimental animals and also in infants, they are able to cure rickets with great speed, ease, and certainty, and to increase very markedly the phosphorus in the blood of infants on a constant diet. When I saw this experimental and clinical work in New York last December, the result had already been reached of demonstrating an annual curve, from month to month, of phosphorus in the blood of infants, with a maximum in June–July, and a minimum in March, following upon the

[1] See the paper by Hess and others in the *Journal of the American Medical Association*, December 30th, 1922.

monthly height of the sun in New York. By radiographic study of the bones of infants, it had also been shown that no new cases of rickets occur in New York in June–July, and the maximum number occur in March. Dr. Hess now informs me that the calcium content of the blood follows the same curve as the phosphorus content. Among earlier noted seasonal effects of sunlight, quoted by Hess in his latest paper, are the presence of increased iodine in the thyroid of cattle from June to November, and the greater resistance of guinea-pigs to aceto-nitrile poisoning in summer.

Hess and his workers have also begun the study of various clothing materials in this connection, and find that they vary in their power of permitting or obstructing the action of light. Specimens of a mercerised cotton, one white and the other black, but otherwise identical, the former allowing light to act and the latter interfering with it, have been examined by me, and I find no difference, due to the black dye, in the spacing between the fibres of the material. But I understand that the Department of Applied Physiology of the Medical Research Council has found, in a series of observations as yet unpublished, that the biological action of light can be graded by temperature. I am glad that these specimens of material are now being studied by the delicate methods associated with the name of Professor Leonard Hill, and think it may be found that the black material produces a higher temperature than the white of the subjacent skin, thus prejudicing those unknown and beneficent chemical reactions which appear to need light and cold for their development. I owe to Professor Leonard Hill the reminder that, many years ago, Sir James Dewar demonstrated the bactericidal action of ultra-violet light upon bacteria *at the surface* of liquid air, but at no deeper level. The action of the light varies according to the temperature factor. The belief grows upon me that the asserted futility of heliotherapy in phthisis is due to the overheating of the patients in the sun. I think that a new chapter will open in the treatment of that disease when practitioners acquaint themselves with the principles and practice of heliotherapy before exposing their patients to the sun.[1]

The power of sunlight and of cod-liver oil in rickets has suggested to Professor Harden that the light may cause the skin to produce vitamin A for itself— though no instance of the synthesis of a vitamin by the animal body is known. The most recent work at the Lister Institute shows that light is unable to replace vitamin A completely, but appears to make a small quantity more effective. Dr. Katherine Coward's work shows that vitamin A is present in the parts of flowers which contain carotene. Sir William Bayliss has suggested to me that the production of this vitamin in green plants is a function of the carotene rather than of chlorophyll, and that probably the carotene acts as a sensitiser for ultra-violet rays. In this connection we must

[1] At Montana Dr. Bernard Hudson, under the influence of Professor Leonard Hill's recent observations on sunlight there, is now exposing *all but the chest* of phthisical patients to the early morning sun, with temperature control.

remember that pigmentation of the skin is a marked feature of the sun-cure, and that patients who do not pigment well do not progress well. No one who has seen and touched the typical pigmented skin of a heliotherapeutic patient can doubt that very active chemical processes are there occurring. Perhaps we should regard the skin less as a mere integument than as an organ of internal secretion. The pigmented skin under the sunlight is surely that; and we may ask whether it contributes, as Sheridan Delépine suggested,[1] to the making of hæmoglobin. I owe also to Sir William Bayliss the information that Dr. H. H. Dale, a member of his committee, has shown that smooth muscle can be made to contract by ultra-violet rays.

Aerial and other photographs of Manchester, and the Potteries, and of Sheffield, taken for me at successive hours on Sunday and Monday, demonstrate the obstruction of sunlight by our urban smoke, the industrial and the domestic chimney being both responsible; but while Sheffield deprives itself of more than half its sunlight, Essen is absolutely smokeless, and Pittsburg, which I have visited for the purposes of this inquiry, has abolished 85 per cent. of its smoke. Sections of the lungs of an agricultural labourer and a typical urban inhabitant of Britain, the latter being heavily infiltrated with smoke, illustrate a cognate aspect of our subject.

Yet another point is illustrated by recent work of Hess, which shows that the milk of cows fed on

[1] *Journal of Physiology*, vol. xii., 1891, p. 27.

pasture in the sunlight maintains the growth and health of young animals, whereas the milk of cows fed in shadow and on vitamin-free fodder will not maintain life. Our children are thus disadvantaged in winter by light-starvation, and by the defect of the milk of light-starved cows.[1]

Photographic study of houses and housing on both sides of the Atlantic illustrates the problem of urban light-starvation. Finding New York smokeless in 1919, I later made investigations with the aid of Dr. Royal S. Copeland, the Health Commissioner of that city, and found that the death rate from pulmonary tuberculosis had been reduced by one-half in the period, 1905–1919, of the operation of the sanitary regulation against smoke.[2] The restoration of sunlight to our urban lives is the next great task of public health in Great Britain.

" There is no darkness but ignorance," as Shakespeare said. In every sense we need " more light." Then we must apply our knowledge, less for heliotherapy than heliohygiene, until we have banished what I call the diseases of darkness, and it may be said of us that " The people that walked in darkness have seen a great light, and they that dwell in the land of the shadow of death, upon them hath the light shined."

[1] To some extent, Antipodean sunlight, in the form of dried milk from New Zealand, comes to the rescue (see Chapter XIII.).

[2] The smoke prohibited in New York or in Winnipeg, where I found similar regulations, need not, as in our futile Public Health Act, be " black." See " The Eugenic Prospect " (Part II., " Let There be Light ") (*loc. cit.*).

CHAPTER III

HIPPOCRATES AND HARLEY STREET

IN the beginning of medicine, Hippocrates practised in the island of Cos. Early in the present century, thanks to the labours of Dr. Rudolph Herzog, of Tübingen, there were brought to light the remains of the great Health Temple of Cos, where the Father of Medicine practised. It was a temple of Æsculapius, son of Phœbus Apollo, god of the sun and medicine and music. The road to the temple from Cos was a sacred way, and the priests were physicians. The Asklepieion, or Health Temple, was about two miles from the sea, at an elevation of about 320 feet, at a point where the range of mountains, which rises on the south coast of Cos to a height of about 2,800 feet, springs from the gentle slopes of the plain. Here, about the year 1903, were discovered the signs which led to the rediscovery of this marvellous place, after twenty-four centuries. In 1906, Dr. Richard Caton, of Liverpool, having visited and studied the labours of the archæologists, bringing to them his medical knowledge, gave a " Friday evening Discourse " [1] at the Royal Institution which I vividly remember, and upon the written form of which I freely draw here.

[1] " Hippocrates and the Newly Discovered Health Temple at Cos," *Proceedings of the Royal Institution*, 1906.

We learn that an effective form of religion was involved in medical practice at that time ; with its prestige, its sanctions, its influence upon the conduct, the conscious and the subconscious mind of the patients ; and of the physicians, let us add, lest we forget a most important factor. Doubtless there were elements of Nature worship in this cult, accounting in some measure for the leading part played by natural means in the practice of the place.

The environmental conditions were exquisite, exhilarating, exalted. Sea and sky, fertile plains and mountains played their part. In this setting, the unequalled architecture of Greece erected a group of noble buildings, which took nothing from Nature, but made her resources better available for man—the proper object of buildings, if I mistake not. As reconstructed in a drawing by Dr. Caton, the main features of this group were three-sided, colonnaded and open stoas, or porticoes, which were instantly brought back to my mind when I visited Queen Mary's Hospital for Children at Carshalton in this inquiry and found that its essential feature, very well shown in photographs from an aeroplane, is a number of three-sided erections, one storey high, which, without architectural beauty, nevertheless are identical in principle with what we find at Cos. We shall not err in applying the term Solarium to the old as well as to the new. Further, we find evidence of an aqueduct and great tanks or basins, doubtless used for the preliminary ceremonial ablutions of the patients—ablutions performed without prejudice to the subsequent extensive use of hydro-therapeutics in many of its forms, a practice in which Hippocrates strongly believed and which was the subject of a *first* series of lectures under the auspices of the University of London as late as 1923. There is some evidence of surgery—as for the reduction of dislocations—and of pharmacy, but drugs were very few and played a very small part in Hippocratic medicine. On the other hand, the utmost importance was attached to diet and to its preparation, cheese and honey being important articles of food in the regimen of the place. As for wine, Hippocrates strongly believed that its tendency, in any quantity, was to weaken rather than invigorate ; but he believed in " water externally, water internally, water eternally," as they say in America nowadays, and there is evidence of several drinking fountains, and one in particular, the sacred spring " of which, no doubt," says Dr. Caton, " every patient was made to drink freely." Especially did anæmic patients drink the " red water," as it was called, from a chalybeate spring higher up in the hills. Finally, remember the palæstra, the large space devoted to gymnastic exercises, of which Dr. Caton writes : " Could we transport ourselves backwards in time to the year 400 B.C., we might have seen in this palæstra such sights as the gouty man casting the discus, walking or running round and round the stoa, or going through the sword or spear exercise, grumbling meanwhile at his prescribed meagre diet, or the weakly and ill-developed youth running, throwing the javelin, or engaging in gentle wrestling, drinking

the 'red water,' and taking a full and rich diet."
But I must leave Dr. Caton and proceed, though not
without quoting his final sentences :

The influence of Hippocrates tended alike to the acqui-
sition of what was new and valuable, and to the denial and
the casting off of all that was useless and superstitious.
While he reverenced the supreme gods, he had more confi-
dence in rest, pure air, exercise, diet, remedies, and in the
restorative powers of Nature than in the interposition of
Asklepios or the influence of the sacred serpents. In fact,
in this building, under the guidance of Hippocrates, medicine
probably arose as a helpful instrumentality, based on
foundations scientific and practical, and in a nobler form
than the world had ever seen, for the relief of the sufferings
of mankind.

We need only add that the Greeks of that age
have never been equalled in body or in mind by any
subsequent peoples in nearly twenty-five centuries.

It was not Harley Street, but its parallel neighbour, Wimpole Street, which Tennyson, in " In
Memoriam," described as the " long, unlovely
street." Both were then, some eighty years ago,
and are still, long and unlovely. They are devoted
to the efforts of the most illustrious students and
servants of life. Not so much as a single blade of
grass is to be found within them ; to that extent,
at least, they illustrate a great aim of modern
surgery, and are sterilised. Except for a good
supply of clean water in the houses, there is no
natural agent of life or health that the medical area
of this mighty metropolis now exhibits. A census
of open windows showed Harley Street houses to
be, for the most part, as nearly hermetically sealed
as those of any other area ; and, since the " air "

is mostly smoke, dried equine excreta and the effluent of motor cars, there is perhaps method in that madness. The rooms are dark and gloomy, and could not be better devised to depress the vital powers and inspire anticipations of the tomb. If it be said that, after all, patients go to Harley Street only for consultations and are treated elsewhere, the reply is that the average nursing home in London—they are not quite so bad, invariably, in the provinces—is an absolute disgrace to every one responsible for it. If one thing is worse than another in these places, after making full allowance for their darkness, their discomfort, their noise, their lack of beauty and cheerfulness, it is perhaps the food and the cooking ; though worst of all, of course, is the abominably mercenary and commercial character of the whole system, as like an Asklepieion as the artificial nightingale in Hans Andersen's story was like the divine singer.

Great Ormond Street Hospital for Sick Children is in need, after seventy-three years' service, and its senior physician, Dr. G. F. Still, a great student, appeals for funds, in order that the hospital may be able to establish a branch in the country. It is just as far from Cos to Great Ormond Street as from Hippocrates to Harley Street. No children's hospital should be in a city, or in any such city as London, apart from the need to provide for accidents and critical emergencies. On one occasion, as I was passing St. George's Hospital with Dr. Rollier, he commented on the fact that we were trying to treat sick people in that building, whilst Hyde Park was unused. Hippocrates would have made the same observation.

The truth is that, like all civilisations before us, ours has run off the rails. With all our getting, we have not got understanding. Our getting includes modern medical science, bacteriology and chemo-therapeutics, of which Hippocrates never dreamed. These things are precious, and he would be a fool who denied it. The daily achievements of the men and women who live in Harley Street—or have rooms there, for most of them live where life is really possible—include many modern miracles, and for these the knife and bottle cult may, in many cases, take full credit. If my teaching here is " back to Hippocrates," I do not mean that we are to abandon carbolic acid and chloroform and thyroid substance, salvarsan and diphtheria antitoxin and " Bayer 205 " and insulin. But I do mean that, whilst we have gained greatly we have lost greatly, in practice, in precept and in principle, and that the medicine of the future will be, as the Father of Medicine would have had it, a practical religion of life, with health temples, for the body and the soul, wherein the true priest and the true physician will serve as one.

CHAPTER IV

VIS MEDICATRIX NATURÆ

TOO often the *vis medicatrix naturæ*, the healing
power of Nature, fails us, and in our need
recourse is had to medicines from without. Until
some fifty years ago, no real knowledge of the causes
of disease existed, and medicines were thus directed
to and valued for the relief of symptoms, which, to
this day, are popularly regarded as diseases, though
most symptoms are, in fact, vital reactions to
disease, and expressions, indeed, of the *vis medicatrix
naturæ*. Many symptoms of beneficent processes
were thus attacked by drugs under a deplorable
misunderstanding, and the pharmacopœia was
immense. Whilst fundamental subjects, such as
psychology, are absent still from the medical curri-
culum, at least in Great Britain, the student con-
tinues to be required to memorise the facts, and
fictions, of hundreds of drugs which have no place
in modern medicine and, in many instances, have
been demonstrated by pharmacology to be inert—
sarsaparilla, for instance, once trusted against
syphilis—or wholly deleterious in any circumstances.
Nevertheless, in this immense and egregious medley
which we have inherited, there was a tiny handful
of drugs of which the last word has yet to be said—
tartar emetic, for instance, which is a salt of

antimony, and quinine and ipecacuanha, discovered by the natives of South America, at dates unknown, to be valuable against malaria and dysentery respectively, and introduced into Europe in the seventeenth century.

Then came Louis Pasteur, whose centenary we recently celebrated, and we learnt that diseases are mostly due to parasites and involve contests for life between the host and the invaders of low degree who have attacked him. Two lines of study were indicated—first, the use of parasiticides, and, secondly, the investigation of the *vis medicatrix naturæ* in the form of immunity, as in natural recovery from an infection. The first and most obvious result was the use of the parasiticide, carbolic acid, by the surgeon, Lister, in what he called antiseptic surgery. Accepted ideas of medication required re-examination in the light of what used to be called the " germ theory " of disease, and the unfortunate fact was discovered that many accepted remedies, and many newly-introduced remedies, were indiscriminate in their deadly action upon living cells, and, whilst they might kill parasitic cells, would also kill the cells of the host, so that it became a toss-up, so to say, which would die first, the " disease " or the patient.

Then came the great creative mind of medicine in this century, Paul Ehrlich, with his concept of " chemo-therapeutics," and his hope of creating or finding drugs which should be as hurtful as possible to parasites and as little hurtful as possible to the organs of the host—" maximally parasitotropic and

minimally organotropic." His work was widely
reviled and libelled here before the war, but already
in 1913, at the last meeting of the International
Medical Congress, he had triumphed, and never in
my life have I seen any man or woman receive such
an ovation as he at St. Thomas's Hospital when he
was to discuss salvarsan. (This is a compound of
arsenic, and good old-fashioned tartar emetic is a
compound of a closely related element, antimony—
a fact worth noting.) His great lecture to the whole
Congress in the Albert Hall on chemo-therapeutics,
which it was also my privilege to hear, laid down the
principles of what we may fairly call the new medicine,
and will doubtless be a classic for ever.

Great triumphs, in every way worthy to set beside
the treatment of syphilis, relapsing fever, yaws, rat-
bite fever, and other infections by spirilla, with
salvarsan or " 606," have been achieved. The
possibilities of arsenic, so combined as to kill spirilla
without killing the tissues of the patient, re-directed
attention to tartar emetic. In the empirical field,
where the profound learning of an Ehrlich and a
high technical equipment in organic chemistry were
not required, some of our own workers, in tropical
and sub-tropical countries, have found some very
happy facts, which already mean life and health
and beauty and joy to immense numbers of persons
who would otherwise be dead or dying or hideous or
miserable. Thanks doubtless to its antimony, tartar
emetic has been found to be a specific against a well-
known tropical disease called kala-azar—the work
of Sir Leonard Rogers being conspicuous here—and

also in the deplorable disease of Egypt and other countries due to infection by the bilharzia worm. No one can say that these results, however, were obtained on the pure principles of chemo-therapeutics or can be explained by them.

Further, it was found that, against one form of dysentery and that alone, due to an invading amœba, ipecacuanha was effective, and that this efficacy resided in its principal alkaloid, long ago called emetine, because of its emetic properties, and a second alkaloid, called cephæline. The pitiful sickness and depression caused by emetine, however, led to the attempt to construct other alkaloids, perhaps by slight modification of emetine, which might be more effective and less distressing. It was found, however, by Dr. H. H. Dale, F.R.S., that, contrary to expectation and to Ehrlich's first principle, other alkaloids, less distressing to the patient, and more potent against the amœba outside the body, were useless clinically, and not until the patient received emetine, with all its toxic symptoms to himself, did he recover.

In a word, the general truth emerges that, often if not always, there is a very marked difference between the action of a drug *in vivo* and *in vitro*, in the living body and in the test tube. Ehrlich himself had shown that salvarsan acts effectively upon spirilla, not by itself but when, for instance, an extract of liver cells is added. In other words, even with the most wonderful and specific and perfectly adapted of drugs, there is needed something done by the body itself for itself. At the moment of the greatest triumphs of artificial therapy the *vis medicatrix naturæ* is found to have " been there all the time," and to be indispensable.

The latest triumph of the chemo-therapeutic principle is the construction, by the German firm of Bayer, of a compound, number 205 in their search of many years, which is a cure, beyond our best hopes, of the deadly and appalling African disease called sleeping-sickness, which is due to a trypanosome, and is not to be confounded with *encephalitis lethargica*, the so-called " sleepy sickness " found in temperate climates. The new remedy is not a dye, but is derived from the trypan-blue of Ehrlich, in his studies against trypanosomes years ago. We shall not be surprised if we learn anon that the vital activities of the patient play an essential part in the cure here also.

Perhaps, in many cases, the tissues act by gradually reducing or oxidising a compound in itself not very toxic, so that tiny quantities of something very potent and effective are gradually produced, exactly where their work is to be done, though to administer so potent a compound directly would be impossible. Some such explanation of many contrasts between action *in vivo* and *in vitro* may serve.

In any case, one sees a general analogy between the reinstatement, so to say, of the *vis medicatrix naturæ* in contemporary chemo-therapeutics and in the various forms of radiotherapy which we are discussing here. When Finsen applied light to lupus, he hoped to kill the tubercle bacilli and cure the patient, just like Ehrlich, at a later date, hoping to kill spirochætes by means of " magic bullets " carrying arsenic. Further inquiry shows that the action of light in reinforcing the *vis medicatrix naturæ* is probably far more important than any mere bactericidal power, and Sonne sees in light a means of so specifically warming the blood that anti-bodies are more easily made in and by it—a direct appeal to the *vis medicatrix naturæ*. Rollier again supposes that the tissues may transform light waves of longer wave-length into ultra-violet rays (presumed to be more bactericidal) in the depths of the body—a parallel to the case of salvarsan or atoxyl, in syphilis or sleeping-sickness, being modified by the tissues, as and where required, so as to produce a specifically toxic agent otherwise as intolerable as would be large doses of ultra-violet light in the blood.

Again, waves of still higher pitch, named after Röntgen, are described as killing malignant cells, and certainly do so, but when the clinicians apply in their patients the lessons taught by experimental radiation of, say, detached and living portions of animal tumours in the laboratory—as now being studied at the Columbia University in New York—they begin to find evidence which, rightly or wrongly, suggests to them that the right dose of Röntgen rays acts no less by stimulating the tissues of the patient than by depressing the enemy cells. Even here, as in the latest developments of chemo-therapy, there may be the indispensable minimum for which we depend upon " ourselves alone " and without which no man can help us.

The teachers of religion proclaim the Divine

mercy, but it will not save, they tell us, unless at least we lift up our hands for it. Without some effort on our part not even omnipotence can save. These matters are far beyond me, but the argument suggests that super-nature is consistent with what I see of nature. The teachers of social science tell us that dribbling coppers to people in gutters, as I have weakly done all my life and always shall do, is futile and unscientific, because these people lack the factor of self-salvation, which is indispensable ; and doubtless this stern doctrine is true. At any rate, it requires some effort to stand in a gutter, I should suppose. Certainly I know that even pre-digested and warmed food will not nourish the body which cannot, at least, put forth the effort to absorb it.

Or, in sum, " God helps those who help themselves." We must accept this principle in relation to the action and uses of sunlight, which ever depend upon our *vital response*.

CHAPTER V

AFTER PASTEUR

ARE we to conclude, in the second century after the birth of Pasteur, that he spoke the last word—even when he said, " It is in the power of man to make all parasitic diseases disappear from the earth " ; or is there more to come, if we will go to meet it ?

As ever, the enlarging sphere of the known finds itself, to use Herbert Spencer's image, in contact with an enlarging surface of the unknown. There is " no end to learning," as Browning's Grammarian knew. The colossal and epoch-making labours of Pasteur, revealing the new world of micro-biology and its relation to the lives of creatures visible to the naked eye, such as ourselves, were not final, but lead the way to new worlds to conquer—not outside but within ourselves. We return from bacteria and bacteriology, with precious conquests, to the proper study of mankind, which is man. The nineteenth century, principally through Pasteur, taught us the main truths about infection ; the twentieth will proceed to new triumphs and truths about nutrition.

The last thing to be inferred from the foregoing is that we have done what we could and should with the work of Pasteur. We have not nearly completed it, in the realm of knowledge, and we have not nearly applied it, in the realm of practice. One of his foremost pupils, Professor Calmette, recently protested, as well he might, against the rebuilding of the devastated area of France with the same shocking lack of primary sanitation that disgraced it before the war ; as if the greatest of Frenchmen had never lived. Heaven knows there is more than enough to be done, in all parts of the world except the newer North American cities, in the direct and obvious application of our knowledge of infection to the conditions of our lives. If that is true of France, or Quebec, or Scotland, what of Bombay or Shanghai ? It will take the rest of our century, no doubt, to persuade mankind that it is worth while to apply the evident teaching of Pasteurism, which any child can understand, to all places where men live. It will take another decade and more, for the matter of that, even to get our dirty and dangerous milk supply in this country pasteurised as it should be. And it will be many years yet before even the Rockefeller Foundation, with its superb sweep of action and its immense resources, can completely wipe yellow fever, for instance, off the face of the earth, as it means to do and doubtless will do. These and a limitless number of further instances might be adduced to show that we are only at the beginning, really, of the translation into happy, healthy human life of the legacy that Pasteur bequeathed us.

Further, a vast amount of work remains to be done in bacteriology proper. We know very little yet about the micro-parasites of many important

to attack. The brain has two hemispheres as the face has two eyes, and though these cannot very well work independently, they serve as indications that the mind must always be used not monocularly but binocularly—to use an analogy first employed, I think, by Dr. John Brown, the author of "Rab and his Friends."

Pasteur's fowl that got its feet wet and that accordingly, its nutrition being disordered, lost its immunity to anthrax bacilli, has everything to teach us. The next great chapter, after Pasteur, as no one knew better than he, is the chapter called Nutrition. During the last few years, in my attempted task of public education, certain subjects have been discussed, and returned to, which fall under this general head. Not very much has been written about bacteriology or its developments, except when some great outstanding achievement required consideration, such as the work of Ehrlich in the formulation of the principles of chemo-therapeutics, and in their application by the construction of salvarsan. But very much has been written about, for instance, vitamins and their relation to growth and health; and about certain radiations, such as those of sunlight in its relation to normal cells, and those named after Röntgen, in their relation to the malignantly altered cells of cancerous growths; and about the "ductless glands" and the "endocrine balance." Generally speaking, I have sought to direct the attention of my readers, and notably of those in Great Britain who have influence in the direction of our national efforts in science, towards the problems of nutrition, not as opposed to but as complementary to, and really even more fundamental than, the problems of infection, upon which nearly all of us in all civilised countries have so properly, naturally and inevitably concentrated our attention during the past half-century, thanks to Pasteur.

We progress in spirals, as Buffon first said. Our movement now brings us back, but at a far higher level, to the point from which the physicians and pathologists before Pasteur were trying, but with a field of vision too circumscribed, to survey the world of health and disease. They thought and wrote much of the "phthisical temperament" or the "tuberculous diathesis," and they used such words as "dyscrasia" to indicate a specific kind of malnutrition that really underlay this or that particular disease. Then came Pasteur, and the talk of dyscrasias and diatheses very naturally began to sound like resounding nonsense. But the study of nutrition and malnutrition is not nonsense; it is fundamental. We are coming back to physiology, with the sure and certain hope of immense gains—such as I have lately been observing for myself in Canada and the United States—added to and in large degree dependent on those things which we owe to Pasteur and the bacteriologists, and which, having proved them all to be very good, we shall evermore hold fast.

CHAPTER VI

THROUGH his closed shutter, as we remember, Newton bored a hole, admitting a ray of "white light," which he broke into a spectrum of colour by means of a prism. "Light is the queen of colours," therefore, as St. Augustine said, and we obtain the conception of a scale or gamut or keyboard or series of notes in what the sun sends us. Further inquiry shows it to consist of an octave of radiations, the violet light pulsating at double the frequency of the red. Already we observe, therefore, that different notes affect our living substance differently, so that in one case we see red, in another green, and in another violet. Already we are in the very depths of the biology and bio-chemistry of light, for we must offer some explanation of colour-vision, and this involves the concept of certain visual substances, situated in the retina, which are specifically acted upon by light of varying frequencies. These chemical compounds, perhaps three or four in number, are presumably acted upon by certain radiations, inducing special excitations of the optic nerve, and their number may correspond to the number of colours we call primary. Hereditary absence of such light-sensitive agents may account for the phenomena of Daltonism or colour-blindness. Here, in this visible octave alone, therefore, we have problems in the specific relation between certain ethereal notes and our living substance, which may occupy the physiologists for decades.

In 1800, however, Herschel went further than Newton, and inserted the bulb of a thermometer in the path of the solar radiation, as broken up by a prism, and found very evident heat effects at a point outside the red light, where to the eye there was nothing. Hence the discovery of the infra-red, or notes of radiant heat, or " heat rays "—badly so-called, since definite heat effects are observed with some of the rays in the visible octave of light. Instead of the thermometer, we may use more subtle means, such as a galvanometer, with a mirror attached, throwing a beam of light on a scale as it rotates under the influence of the electricity induced by even infinitesimal measures of heat ; and here, also, we find a whole realm of physical fact, in parallel with the octave of light, and profoundly important in its biological connections. Thus, we note that these rays of lower pitch and longer wave-length do not affect the chemical substances of the retina ; and, so long ago as 1779, it was shown by Ingenhouss that it is the visible light rays and not the heat rays of the sun that so act upon the chlorophyll of the green leaf as to effect the dissociation of carbon dioxide—the primary chemical act upon which the entire living world depends. This elementary distinction between the chemical meanings and potencies of the light and the heat of the sun respectively has been ignored with calamitous consequences as recently as our own time.

Contemporary physicists have demonstrated the existence and studied the properties of about nine octaves of these infra-red or " dark heat rays " : an astonishing extension, in itself, of the single octave of visible light.

Only a year later than Herschel, Ritter and Wollaston showed that rays having chemical power were situated in the region beyond the violet. They would blacken silver chloride, these ultra-violet, " photographic," " chemical," or " actinic " rays, and their upward range is also surprising. We can study them in the solar radiation and also in artificial light, notably that produced by passing an electric current through mercury vapour in a vacuum bounded by quartz, through which, unlike ordinary glass, these rays of short wave-length can pass. Thus we can recognise no fewer than three octaves of the ultra-violet spectrum, and can distinguish different parts of it according to their physico-chemical properties.

At this point we may compare artificial sources of radiation with what reaches us from the sun, and we obtain the idea that the atmosphere is a selective filter, allowing certain parts only of the solar radiation to reach us—the visible octave and certain notes above and below it. We are to regard man as a being evolved to fit and thrive in the conditions of his environment, the " *milieu environnant*," in the classical phrase of Lamarck, and therefore we need not be surprised to learn that the higher pitched notes of the ultra-violet spectrum would be distinctly noxious to our bodies if they were not screened from us by the atmospheric ocean at the bottom of which we live. On the other hand, the lower notes of the ultra-violet, next to the visible violet itself, are unquestionably necessary for our lives, and we suffer when, by any artificial means, we interfere with the selective action of the atmosphere, and exclude the lower as well as the higher ultra-violet notes. In a communication to *Nature*,[1] *àpropos* my demand for a systematic inquiry into this subject, Sir Oliver Lodge quoted certain thirty-year-old experiments made by himself and the late Professor Marshall Ward, which demonstrated the antiseptic action upon pathogenic bacteria of ultra-violet rays of just those wave-lengths which are arrested by the addition of coal-smoke to the beneficent filter of air above our cities.

When the late Professor Wilhelm von Röntgen discovered the rays to which he gave the name, no longer applicable, of X, they seemed to be far apart from all other natural phenomena. It is no longer so. The Röntgen rays are themselves part of the invisible spectrum ; they are doubtless sent us by the sun, but mercifully arrested by the atmosphere, and they can be measured and placed upon the ethereal scale like any others. Until quite recently there remained a large gap between the three octaves of the ultra-violet and the seven octaves of the Röntgen rays, but that gap has now been filled in, and we may call the ethereal keyboard continuous,

[1] December 15th, 1921.

from the visible spectrum upwards through the ultra-violet even to the so-called gamma rays produced by radium and other radio-active substances—rays of extreme frequency and shortness, the latter represented by such a figure as one ten-millionth of a millimetre.

The action of these high-pitched rays upon living matter is marked, characteristic and important. It is also obscure and paradoxical, for by them morbid growths may be caused and morbid growths may be killed. In general, they must be called destructive to living matter, and we must be grateful to the atmosphere for screening them from us. Nevertheless, the ethereal organ is, in my view, a part of nature upon which the intelligence of man is to play, and I doubt not that, in one way or another, every note in the gamut, singly or in combination, can be used for the purposes of man. Nothing in the records of the fight against malignant disease hitherto surpasses the results obtained by the use of those highest notes of the ethereal gamut which we call the gamma rays of radium.[1]

Below the nine octaves of the " infra-red " or "dark heat rays " there is at present an unfilled gap of some four octaves, the radiations in which have still to be discovered. Below that we can identify some twelve octaves of Hertzian waves, and further still another twelve octaves or so of similar waves, unknown to Hertz, which are now in wide use for the purposes of " wireless " and " broadcasting."

[1] See, for instance, the invaluable and most hopeful Report for 1922 of the Radium Institute, Riding House Street, W.

By the time we reach the longest of these, the wave-length becomes immense and may be measured in miles, perhaps as many as ten. Here, also, is an immense range of notes, which may be touched in the service of man.

During his Christmas lectures,[1] " adapted to a juvenile auditory," at the Royal Institution in 1921, continuing that unbroken series of more than three-quarters of a century which began with the genius and initiative of Faraday himself, Professor J. A. Fleming had a long narrow diagram pinned right across the back wall of the theatre. He called it " The Keyboard of the Electric Wave Organ," and upon it was indicated a total of fifty octaves, of which nearly the whole were known at that date, and the gaps have very nearly disappeared altogether to-day. How insignificant, almost, in that long range, was the fiftieth part of it, one tiny multi-coloured octave, which we call light, because our eyes are so made as to be chemically affected by it ! And what an achievement for physics, for a handful of men working with meagre resources, during a century or two, to have found and studied an almost unbroken sequence of radiations, of which Newton's spectrum is only a fiftieth part !

Amongst the vast and fascinating problems of the

[1] Professor Fleming has now published an amplified and well-illustrated revision of those admirable lectures in a volume entitled " Electrons, Electric Waves, and Wireless Telephony " (The Wireless Press, Ltd., 12 and 13, Henrietta Street, Strand, W.C.). Professor Fleming's invention of the thermionic valve and his power of exposition make his volume invaluable as authority and guidance for " wireless " amateurs. This chapter merely deals with a single point in its general aspect.

immediate future are all those which are concerned with the relations between this mighty gamut and the chemistry of living things. The most remarkable and beneficent achievements of contemporary medical science, covering an immense field of pathology, depend entirely upon this relation, only the barest rudiments of which have yet been touched by workers in any field. The remarkable new work of Professors Baly and Heilbron in the University of Liverpool carries our knowledge of photo-synthesis a stage further, elucidating the processes by which certain parts of the solar radiation effect the construction, in the green leaf, of a special kind of formaldehyde, which is the forerunner of the carbohydrates, the starches and sugars ; whilst the earlier stages of the synthesis of proteins by the same mechanism can now be traced.

Meanwhile, they are telephoning across the Atlantic by the use of the lowest notes of the ether wave organ, whilst even cancer of the tongue is beginning to yield to the notes of highest pitch. We may envy the organists of the future, with such an instrument to play upon.

CHAPTER VII

MODERN SUN-WORSHIP

1. Its Creed

THE light of day is the source of all life. It is conceivable that, at some remote age, before the solar radiations could penetrate through the earth's then dense atmosphere, terrestrial radiant energy may have served the needs of living things, but in our own time all the energy that flows through all living bodies, vegetable and animal, including even those of the ocean depths, where no light can penetrate, is the transmuted light of day. It is, of course, possible to have too much of a good thing, and there is, for instance, a disease known as sun-stroke, though very few cases so called are really sun-stroke at all, the greater number being more properly called heat-stroke, a wholly different thing. It is true, also, that, especially if one's youth were spent, say, in Scotland, one may weary of the sun of California. But, in general, light is the creator of our lives and their chief stimulant. When the light fails, or even when we shut our eyes, we tend to go to sleep, and the diurnal-nocturnal rotation is beneficent.

The colours of life, which are green and red with their derivatives, are products of the light, and use the light. The cellar-grown plant cannot produce chlorophyll, nor the cellar-grown child enough hæmoglobin, and it is the chlorophyll by means of which the solar energy dissociates carbon dioxide, returning the oxygen to the air, keeping the carbon, adding it to water obtained through the root, and producing (as has now been experimentally demonstrated) formaldehyde, CH_2O, the formula of which, if we multiply it, gives us a fair idea of the typical carbohydrates, starch and glucose, $C_6H_{10}O_5$ and $C_6H_{12}O_6$, of which the latter is the sugar of our blood, and the former is one of our foodstuffs, which appropriate ferments, produced by the salivary glands and the pancreas, are ready to convert into the latter.

The skin is sensitive to light. In many animals— and the body of man is certainly an animal—the skin contains many cells in which pigment is formed under the action of light, and in some instances the pigment of these cells can be observed to alter its condition in the presence of light. Thus, by what evolutionary process is not our present question, has been evolved the eye, wherein the general cutaneous sensibility to light is most superbly specialised and a stimulant effect of that agent is most particularly achieved.

This, however, is not to say that the general cutaneous surface is not affected by light. The phenomenon called sun-burn, which we observe more especially in brunettes, who have a larger measure of pigment and pigment-forming power in their skin cells, illustrates the sensibility of the skin to light, and so, less beautifully, do the freckles which we observe under the same influence in blondes, being very common, for instance, in Scotland, which contains the fairest inhabitants of our islands—that is to say, those whose skin cells have the least pigment and pigment-forming power.

The evidence of the lakes and the mountains in Switzerland, however, shows that blondes are by no means incapable of developing pigment without freckles. On the Lake of Geneva you may see heads of hair so blonde as to look almost white, and light blue eyes, going with skins which have tanned an even hue, deeper than copper. We must assume, therefore, that the incapacity of the blonde Scot, as a rule, to tan properly under the sun is not a necessary condition of his skin. Very probably, where the sun really shines and goes on shining, as at Geneva he would cease to freckle, and would tan like the fair-haired, blue-eyed, copper-skinned blondes who here attract the speculation of the eye and the mind. The question arises, Can a copper-skinned person be a blonde ? Or, when we talk of Nature or heredity as determining certain characters, are we not always assuming certain conditions of nurture or environment ? Polar explorers record that, after prolonged absence of sunlight, all the eyes of their men are blue. The brown pigment can be developed only in the presence of light. Are such brown-eyed men really blue-eyed, as these copper-coloured swimmers are fair skinned ? And, finally, how sure are we that persistent exposure to intense sunlight, after some generations, may not transform the racial colour of the skin—I will not say at birth, for the new-born negro skin, not yet exposed to light, though descended from parents whose skins have been so exposed, is scarcely black ? A few years ago such a question, at least in England, though not in France or America, would have been thought heretical, but recent advances in experimental evolution make it impossible to dismiss the neo-Lamarckians with a gesture, or with the remark that no conceivable mechanism exists for such a process as they postulate.

We note in passing that this power of the skin, whilst it doubtless indicates a nervous response to light and enables us to guess how light may thus affect the whole body through the nervous system, also indicates that the blood must be protected from excessive radiations. The presence of pigment affords this protection, and thus we have a very simple explanation of the general fact that the density of skin pigmentation in mankind between the Poles and the Equator is in direct proportion to the intensity of the radiations to which we are exposed. It behoves us also to remember, for the better understanding of certain wonderful facts in modern therapeutics, that radiations, whilst necessary for life, may, in excess and under certain conditions, be deadly to living cells. The proposition may also be hazarded that cells of low, simple and primitive type—as, for instance, the red cells of the blood, bacteria and the cells of malignant growths—are specially susceptible to radiations. (This may not be true—I used the word " hazarded " advisedly.

We do not know, for instance, what the direct effect of light would be upon the cells of the cerebral cortex, which are the highest that we know ; but the generalisation is useful as a working hypothesis.)

We have, then, in light, generally speaking, a supreme agent of life and death, with direct and profound influences of various kinds upon all forms of life—not least through the eye upon the brain of man. We must ask the physicists to tell us all they can about it. Briefly, as we know, we may use the analogy of the keyboard of a piano. There are those nowadays who suggest that it may be necessary to revive in modified form the " particulate " or " corpuscular " theory of light which was held by Newton. But we may be content here to think in terms of ethereal waves, and then we will say, as we saw in the previous chapter, that the light which our eyes can see corresponds to something like the middle octave of a piano keyboard, whilst above and below it are radiations none the less real though invisible. Downwards through the infra-red and heat rays we proceed, the number of vibrations per second becoming less frequent and the wavelengths longer, until, they say, we reach the electrical waves of wireless telegraphy, the wavelengths of which may be half a mile or more. (Our visible octave, we may remember, is an electro-magnetic phenomenon according to Clerk-Maxwell.) Many of these vibrations are of great therapeutic interest in various forms of electrical treatment which will not here be discussed. In the other direction we pass through the actinic or ultra-violet rays, with their very marked

influence upon the chemicals of a photographic plate
and upon living things, and then, it may be, after
traversing many octaves, we imagine ourselves arriv-
ing at the Röntgen rays, so-called soft and hard, with
their very marked effects upon living tissues and
cells—amongst which we may remark the power,
under certain conditions respectively, of killing some
malignant cells, of causing malignant growths, of
killing such fungi as that of ringworm, and of killing
the " germ-plasm " and thus causing sterility in
persons long exposed to them. The various actions
of radium must be remembered in parallelism with
those of the Röntgen rays.

A brief survey such as the foregoing shows that
there must be great and varied possibilities for
medicine (i.e., healing) in the use of light of various
kinds in various ways, and it is certainly true that
during the present century the science of phototherapy, as we may most generally call it, has made
great conquests, and may claim a place beside that
form of medicine which consists in the administration
of what the public calls " medicine." And it would
remarkably appear that the line of progress is from
extremely artificial applications of light to its more
natural uses, now known as heliotherapy, and
ultimately from any kind of therapeutics to prophy-
laxis—which we may call helio-hygiene, or scientific
or modern sun-worship, as the reader pleases.

2. ITS HISTORY

Omitting a few names worthy of mention, we
must proclaim a young Dane, Dr. Niels R. Finsen, a

leading pioneer in the practice of modern sun-worship. He was working at the subject in the last decade of the nineteenth century, asking such questions as whether, if the actinic or chemical rays of the spectrum be favourable to chemical changes, the victim of small-pox may not be benefited by protection from such rays, in the hope that, exposed only to red light, the pustules may not be so grave in their development. It is probably of only historical interest to recall those experiments. But later, not forgetful of the demonstration by Koch and others that light is antiseptic to the tubercle bacillus, Finsen began to attempt the cure of lupus, a form of cutaneous tuberculosis, by means of light, and obtained results much superior to those of the knife or any other surgical instrument. It was, and still widely is, believed that the ultra-violet rays are the most useful, and hence various steps have been taken in order either to filter sunlight or to use artificial light which is rich in the rays of shorter wavelength. The red rays and heat rays are hot and burning, and perhaps not therapeutic, and, in any case, they would burn so severely that the patient must be protected from them. Thus, in the earlier forms of photo-therapeutics, not yet really natural in the sense in which that word may be applied to the greatest work now being done to-day, we recall that the patients were exposed in one instance and on one theory to red light only, and in another instance and on another theory to light from the other end of the spectrum. But we shall see whether the whole of the sunlight through and in which our species has been evolved is not generally better for us, in disease and in health, than any of its parts.

Where sunlight is not available artificial light must be used, and we may choose our light in accordance with any theory we may hold as to the relative value of various parts of the spectrum. Hence, in Finsen's work, which earned for him, shortly before his premature death, the Nobel Prize in Medicine, the local use of concentrated sunlight was replaced by that of artificial light rich in the higher-pitched rays to which special virtue is supposed to be attached.

London owes much to Queen Alexandra for her interest in the work of her young fellow countryman, whereby the Finsen treatment for lupus was early installed at the London Hospital, where many cases of this disease were and still are to be found. After several years of observation of surgery in the treatment of local tuberculosis, a profound impression was made upon me, by nature a modern Zoroastrian, when I visited the " London " more than twenty years ago and saw the Finsen light in action. Very intense radiations are focussed on the patch of disease for a certain period daily, passing through a double lens of quartz, between the parts of which cold water circulates, absorbing the heat rays. The results are admirable. By light and light alone, the patient is usually cured, with a minimum of scarring, deformation or destruction of healthy tissues. We note that the light does not penetrate far, and that the shortest rays are those which are most quickly absorbed. When we look at the tip of the ear, beyond which a bright white light shines, and see it red, we realise that, whilst red light may come through the blood, the rays of higher pitch are absorbed. If, therefore, we desire to obtain the healing action of those rays at any appreciable depth, we must press the skin very firmly, so as to keep out of it the blood which would otherwise absorb the rays and prevent them from doing their work except at the very shallowest levels.

Influenced, no doubt, by the valuable demonstrations of Koch, Finsen believed that the light with which he cured lupus acted as a parasiticide, an antiseptic which killed the tubercle bacilli and allowed the patient's tissues to heal accordingly. Then the question arises whether, in fact, the light may not work rather as a stimulant to the defending tissues than as lethal to the invaders. This question, whilst of high scientific interest, is not merely academic and irrelevant to practice. Our answer to the question how light cures is of high practical importance. The answer, I believe, is that the Finsen light cures—in chief, at least—by helping the tissues to help themselves, and hence we may guess that light may cure even when it cannot possibly reach the tubercle bacilli in order to exercise any antiseptic action upon them ; and thereupon we may begin to use light upon the body generally, for the cure of local conditions, not only superficial, such as lupus, but however deeply seated. And when we do so, we modern sun-worshippers are rewarded beyond our most sanguine dreams, as by a deity who answers prayer beyond all that we can ask or think.

But, for the moment, let us pursue the truth that light, or certain kinds of light, may be directly destructive to our enemies of various kinds. Along this line much may be done, even though it be nothing to what may be done on the subtler and less comprehensible assumption. Thus, we may seek certain exceptional kinds of radiation—the more novel, exceptional and remarkable the better our patients will be pleased—and try to obtain from them results which, it goes without saying, no one would expect from ordinary daylight. And we are certainly rewarded up to a point. Certain of the Röntgen rays, for instance, called "hard," have a high penetrative power and are directly lethal to living cells, and to different kinds of cells in different degree. The best resources of the physicists must be invoked in order to make available for the clinician the most precise doses of rays of the most definite wavelength, and invaluable advances have very recently been made in this respect. Clinical results improve *pari passu*, and we cannot but believe that greater things than hitherto—and those are well worth while—will yet be achieved in the control of malignant cells by the action of this invisible light.

In the same category note the radiations from radium. Certain of these rays have a definitely selective action upon living cells. In the least malignant and most superficial form of malignant disease, known as rodent ulcer, radium acts " like a charm." I am not a practitioner of any branch of medicine or surgery, but it was lately my duty to take an elderly friend to a dermatologist, who sent her to the Radium Institute,[1] where her cheek was once exposed to radium, unscreened, for an hour and a half, and was perfectly cured, without pain and with a result, from the æsthetic point of view, otherwise utterly unobtainable. Of course, such achievements are splendid in themselves and rich in promise of much more along the same lines. The reader who wishes to learn more about radium-therapy should obtain the reports of the Radium Institute, and he will then realise how much we owe to the late King Edward for his influence in founding the Institute, and how much we shall owe to Madame Curie, now in Paris with the 100,000 dollars' worth of radium which was lately given to her by the women of America. But I am inclined to believe that the best services rendered by Professor William Röntgen, by the late Professors Finsen and Pierre Curie and by Madame Curie to modern therapeutics consist less in the healing powers of the radiations from a Crookes tube, a Finsen lamp, or from radium, than in the demonstration that any radiations may have such powers.

From these exceedingly rare, artificial forms of radio-therapeutics, demonstrated to be potent, we are entitled to proceed to the plain everyday use of the light of the sun, nor can any one say that our hopes are "high-fantastical" or contrary to anything in already recorded experience. Indeed, are we not entitled to say that, if Röntgen rays and the radiations of radium or of its emanation are in certain conditions sanative and therapeutic, though neither of

[1] Riding House Street, Langham Place, London.

these have any natural relation to mankind, it is *a priori* immeasurably more probable that sunlight itself, part of the natural environment of man, will be sanative and therapeutic ? Let us state the truth as it appears to-day. It is that, when we have added together all the healing and healthful virtues of the Finsen light and radium and the Röntgen rays, and all the uses of heat rays in, for instance, the local treatment of rheumatism at Harrogate or elsewhere, and all the uses of electrical waves in the care of atrophied or unused muscles, or in any other respect ; that is, when every particular form of radiation from one end of the ethereal gamut—if that is what it be— to the other has been tried and exploited to the uttermost, even including all and every advance that may yet be hoped for in the attack on malignant cells— the value of natural sunlight upon us children of light, whether as therapeutic in certain forms of disease, such as so-called surgical tuberculosis, or as hygienic and prophylactic during developmental years, and maturity and old age, outweighs all these other things as the Atlantic outweighs the contents of the *Olympic's* swimming bath. Until seeing Leysin I could not have written thus, even though I have been proclaiming the value of light all my life. It is the cliniques of Dr. Rollier at Leysin, in Switzerland, that have really opened eyes which I had already thought to be wide open to the value of light.

The truth is that we are Naamanites one and all. Perhaps we admire Pasteur, who said that " *Tout est miracle* " and Walt Whitman, who wrote superbly

about natural miracles in more poems than one ; and
we proclaim the value of simple daily things ; but
the moment that some surprising novelty is
announced we forget ourselves and our philosophy—
like the great crowd of doctors who had listened to
a lecture on X-ray therapeutics at a medical congress
a few years ago, and who promptly walked out of the
lecture theatre when Dr. Rollier followed with a
paper on mere heliotherapy. Naaman the leper
wanted thaumaturgy, some marvellous recitation, or
passes of the hands, or invocations of Heaven, and
he was told to "wash and be clean." What an
insult ! What banality ! We want a buzzing X-ray
tube, a good bedside manner, a superb operating
theatre, a perfectly modelled plaster of Paris jacket,
a drug with a high number, a long name and a
remarkable history, like 606, or anti-tuberculosis
serum made at vast expense by the inoculation of
animals ; and when, as Elisha long ago told the
leprous to strip and bathe in the water of common
Jordan and be clean, Rollier now tells the tuberculous
to strip and bathe in the light of common day and
be well, we think his formula too simple—simpletons
that we are.

3. Its High Priest and His Temple

Postponing theory, let us seek the sun and place
therein our ill folk whom we have hitherto failed to
cure with our best efforts of surgery and medicaments.
In certain common and chronic diseases, notorious
especially throughout the temperate zones, we
achieve results unapproachable by any other means.

The high priest of modern sun-worship is Dr. A. Rollier, and his temple is Leysin, in Switzerland. There are many other places now where heliotherapy is practised on his lines. Some are in the mountains, as Leysin is, some are on the sea. The question of altitude is very interesting and must be discussed. But here we may briefly describe Leysin, with the explicit premise that no peculiar virtues inhere in this place, that in some respects it may be inferior to many other places which might be and are not used for heliotherapy, such as California in especial, and that the therapeutic lessons of Leysin are of supreme importance, not at all in themselves, but because of the prophylactic lessons they teach, for our cities, homes, schools, workshops or mines, wherever they may be.

Leysin is a little place at an altitude of 1,450 metres in the Alpes Vaudoises. It is admirably sheltered from the north wind, and has long been a resort of consumptives. There, for personal reasons, it happened that Dr. Rollier began to practise his profession and to attempt the systematic use of the sun-cure in 1903. That is a long time ago, and here am I discussing the subject of heliotherapy as if it were a new discovery. If work like this had been done in the United States, it would be a household word, millionaire philanthropists would have endowed it galore, and it would have been copied everywhere. But it was done by a quiet man in a small country, and though visitors from afar have been to see his work and its lovely results, the Prometheus-Æsculapius of Leysin is still almost

unknown, even in the professional circles that are
concerned with tuberculosis. After an interval of
many years, the International Congress Against
Tuberculosis met again in London in 1921. Nothing
connected with heliotherapy was on the programme.
In 1913 Rollier came to the great International
Medical Congress in London and read a paper,
showing lantern slides and some kinema films.
There were about twenty doctors present and none
of them, he thinks, were English. What astonishes
me is that no American has found out this open
secret and made fame and fortune for himself, years
ago, in California. It is true that Rollier's books—
with one exception, in 1923—are not to be had in
English, and that the first was published in the first
year of the war ; but to-day, in many parts of the
world, tuberculosis is a more formidable problem
than ever before, and no excuse remains for the
neglect of the proven natural remedy and preventive.
This is notably so in France, where the Rockefeller
Foundation and the American Red Cross have been
doing anti-tuberculous work since the war.

Apart from theory, however, all we need to know
is to be found in Rollier's works, to which the
reference is given below.[1]

At the present time Rollier's patients number

[1] " La Cure de Soleil," 1914, 20 francs ; " L'Ecole au Soleil," 1915,
1.50 francs ; " Le Pansement Solaire : Héliothérapie de certaines
affections chirurgicales et des blessures de guerre," 1916, 1.50 francs,
obtainable from Payot & Co., Lausanne ; and " Comment lutter
contre la Tuberculose ? " 1919, a small, but very valuable, brochure,
obtainable from J. A. Sauvain, Librairie des Frènes, Leysin. (The
francs are Swiss). " La Cure de Soleil " has been rewritten and
published in English under the title of " Heliotherapy," 1923.

nearly a thousand, disposed in some thirty-seven cliniques, which are built with balconies facing the sun. Two of these cliniques are maintained by the Swiss Government for the treatment of its soldiers. There are cliniques for poor patients also.

The patients are, of course, breathing pure air, receiving fresh food, free from chance of further infection, and provided with the apparatus of orthopædic surgery in general. Also they enjoy whatever advantages follow from living at a high altitude. We have to ask, What are the essential factors of their cure ? The answer is that, whilst other factors aid, and none should be neglected, the sunlight is *the* therapeutic agent. To breathe pure air, instead of city air contaminated with the products of the combustion of coal, is doubtless an advantage. To be away from massive and repeated infection is an advantage ; perhaps that is the chief boon of open-air treatment as such. The diet is remarkably unremarkable. Dr. Rollier regards the sun as the best stimulant. He discards meat, except very rarely, and absolutely excludes alcohol in all stages of all cases. He told me that it was much easier to feed his poor patients properly ; those who paid suspected him of trying to make money out of them when he fed them as simply as he desires. Cereals and milk and its products and vegetables and fruit are relied on. Cod-liver oil is not used. This was disconcerting to me until I remembered what an abundance of vitamin A the patients must receive in the fresh vegetable leaves which they consume so freely. Overfeeding, hitherto a cardinal principle in the therapeutics of tuberculosis, Rollier detests and scrupulously avoids. The clinical evidence is clear that, when the sunlight fails, as it not infrequently does at Leysin, the patients are injured, and that they prosper when it returns. The natural process of excretion of rubbish—such as a morsel of dead bone—may be observed to cease in obscure weather, and be resumed when the process of insolation is again permitted by the atmospheric conditions.

Now the physicists tell us that the violet and ultra-violet rays of light are those which exert chemical action, both upon photographic salts and upon living things. These rays it is which cause the amusingly extreme pigmentation of Rollier's patients, and his general view is that patients who do not pigment well do not recover well. We know, further, that these actinic rays, and the actinic power of light accordingly, tend to diminish more rapidly than the rest of sunlight as it descends to the earth. In his work on "The Sun," the American astronomer, Abbot, shows experimentally that the light at, say, the height of Leysin, is much more abundant in these precious rays than at sea level. This is of immense practical importance presumably. Are we to say that, for such results in cure and prevention as Leysin achieves, we must necessarily go some 5,000 feet or so up into the sky ? If so, whilst this work remains of immense scientific interest, and whilst we must everywhere possible provide such places as Leysin, the general prospects for mankind are much diminished, and especially my own interest, in the application of modern sun-worship to everyday urban hygiene, receives a serious check. But, first, let it be averred that every argument for the special value of the violet and ultra-violet rays is an argument against those particles of coal-smoke which selectively absorb those very rays. The glorious red sunsets of smoky London, which delighted Rodin, owe their colour to the fact that the abominable dirt of the atmosphere retains the most precious elements of the light—especially, of course, when the rays, at sunset, are falling obliquely and therefore have more dirt to penetrate—and allow the red rays, which are longer, but less valuable, to pass through.

Fortunately, we have English evidence which proves that the " climate of altitude " is not essential for the sun-cure ; or, in other words, if our belief as to the primary value of the actinic rays be correct, that enough of such rays may reach us, even at sea level, if the atmosphere be unpolluted by smoke. This evidence is to be found in the records of the Lord Mayor Treloar Cripples' Hospital and College, Alton, Hants. The student may be referred to its publications and also to a recent paper [1] by Sir Henry Gauvain, M.D., its Medical Superintendent. Admirable results are also obtained at Berck, in France, at the sea level. Not much am I interested to decide whether the low or the high altitude is preferable. The all-important fact is that, at any level at which we human beings live, enough of the sanative and therapeutic part of sunlight may reach us for the cure of disease and the preservation of

[1] *The Lancet*, 1921, i., 1065 : " The Non-Operative Treatment of Surgical Tuberculosis."

health. In this study of the subject, I am concerned
to suggest not that Leysin has any unique properties,
but that what is done there may be, indeed is, being
done at sea level, and is of immediate relevance to
the possibilities of, say, Cornwall and California.

The patient is cured by the action of light on the
skin. After a day at Leysin, one gains an entirely
new respect for the skin. Generally speaking,
Rollier exposes the new patient's feet for five
minutes twice or thrice the first day, for ten the
second day and so on; the legs for five minutes
twice or thrice the second day, ten the third and so
on; until after about a fortnight the entire body is
exposed for from three to six hours daily. He
cannot expect the skin to respond until it has had
a chance. This admirable organ, the natural
clothing of the body, which grows continuously
throughout life, which has at least four absolutely
distinct sets of sensory nerves distributed to it,
which is essential in the regulation of the temperature, which is waterproof from without inwards,
but allows the excretory sweat to escape freely,
which, when unbroken, is microbe-proof, and which
can readily absorb sunlight—this most beautiful,
versatile and wonderful organ is, for the most part,
smothered, blanched and blinded in clothes, and
can only gradually be restored to the air and light
which are its natural surroundings. Then, and only
then, we learn what it is capable of.

Properly aired and lighted, the skin becomes a
velvety, supple, copper-coloured tissue, absolutely
immune from anything of the nature of pimples or

acne, incapable of being vaccinated, and its little hairs usually show considerable development. When the visitor touches such a skin, in the cool air, he is surprised to find it quite warm. The sun was not shining when I did so first, and the patient was, of course, perfectly nude except for a loin-cloth. Evidently plenty of heat was somehow being produced in that little body, with so large a surface to cool by, relatively to its mass. This would seem to be a puzzle, for these patients have, in many instances, never moved a muscle—practically speaking—for months ; they have not even had their muscles innervated by the faradic current ; they have not been massaged. But always the muscles are firm and well-developed under the warm skin. " The sun is the best masseur," said Dr. Rollier to me ; and one realises that the stimulant light, playing upon the nude skin in the cool air, induces and maintains that condition of tone in the muscles which, indeed, moves no joints but is yet a form of muscular activity essential for the production of bodily heat and for the proper posture of the bodily parts. Hence we understand how plaster of Paris apparatus is here as utterly unknown as the knife. The tone of the muscles, thanks to the nude skin and the reflex response to the light, is enough to keep the recovering young spine, for instance, in proper position, and to form what Rollier calls the " *corset musculaire*." One sees very little fat on any of the patients. Their condition is more like that of the trained athlete, and one's ideas as to the importance of fat in tuberculosis go by the board.

The Greeks believed in stripping the skin, and when we speak of gymnastics we refer to that practice. The idea that a nude person, with pigmented and properly functioning skin, is not clothed soon leaves one at Leysin. Also conventional ideas of modesty receive their death-blow. On this point Dr. Rollier writes very interestingly in his " Ecole au Soleil," where he has to consider the effect of denudation upon the ideas and conduct of his children, and of their parents, and I wish particularly to direct the attention of American readers to this matter. The ideas of decency which, both in the United States and Canada, require that a girl, when bathing, shall wear stockings " of full length "— lest her knees be visible—and which compel a visitor to don a local suit, cumbrous for swimming, because his own " university costume," brought from home, is insufficiently proper—require re-examination in the light of many sciences, abstract and concrete, from ethics to heliotherapy. Our present attitude to the skin is a stupid and dangerous insult to the light of day and to the human body, and, like other blasphemies against " *Cosmos sive Deus*," as Spinoza would have said, is duly visited upon us.

The exposure to light greatly increases the circulation through the now well-nourished skin. It causes pigmentation, the result of which is to effect the still more complete absorption of the ultra-violet rays. In any case these rays are very quickly stopped by the skin, as by coal-smoke in the air, whilst the red rays pass on. Dr. Rollier suggests that the ultra-violet rays may be transformed by the pigment into red rays, of greater penetration, and quotes evidence to show that red rays are antiseptic. The curative action of the light, even at some depth, might thus be accounted for. For myself, I think no explanation yet afforded to be adequate. Processes vastly more subtle than the killing of bacilli by radiations are at work, as we see by the value of the light, generally applied to the skin, upon deep-seated local infections, and by the curative results of heliotherapy in many affections which no one believes to be of microbic origin.

Also the skin, or, rather, the blood abundantly moving through the superficial capillaries, absorbs much of the light and retains it. The physics and the physiology of this matter are still obscure, but the evidence we possess, and especially the work of Sonne at the Finsen Medical Light Institute in Copenhagen, is to the effect that the radiant energy must count as part of the energy of the body. There is so much less need to burn up fats or carbohydrates in order to keep the blood warm, if heat is directly passing into it by the skin. Thus, the light is a skin food, in one sense of that term, and saves the digestive mechanism—so that the very moderate dietary of Leysin can be understood. These patients, perhaps in considerable degree, are living directly on light, as green plants do, and are not in so much need of feeding upon the food which green plants have thus made.

And, however it be, the patient loses first his pain and then his fever—a few days and both are done, and thereafter he proceeds to recover. If he arrived with pus in some cavity, it may be withdrawn by puncture, but all " surgery " is ended. " Surgical tuberculosis " is a term which should be regarded as belonging to and ending with the nineteenth century. The knife in these cases is a barbaric and dangerous anachronism. Leysin and other places where heliotherapy is practised constitute the utter condemnation of all places throughout the world where surgeons operate for tuberculous glands in the neck or " white swellings," or any other form of tuberculosis. Their very best results, rarely enough attained, are destructive, mutilative, crippling, hideous, compared with the everyday miracles of heliotherapy.

What, then, ought we to do about it, or, in Dr. Rollier's phrase, " *Comment lutter contre la tuberculose* ? "

4. Its Rewards and Warnings

The rewards of the modern sun-worshipper are the prevention and cure of what I have here and elsewhere, in previous years, called the " diseases of darkness." Of these tuberculosis is the most deadly, by far ; the tubercle bacillus is the " captain of the men of death," as Osler called him, or " the prince of the powers of darkness," as I would call him ; the destruction effected by this disease, which should be unknown, is appalling, and our present methods of dealing with it are pitifully inadequate. In a previous volume I have discussed the desolating records of our sanatoria in Great Britain in this respect. But many other diseases belong to the same category.   Wholly or in part I include rickets, our general urban anæmia, and many pulmonary infections amongst the diseases of darkness. At Leysin these diseases are unknown. There is no bronchitis, there are no colds in the head, there is no rheumatism. Rollier has perhaps one development of tuberculous meningitis in a year, among all the advanced and ghastly cases that come to him. His records of customary success, during twenty years, include many extreme cases of spinal tuberculosis, with paralysed lower limbs, and so forth, tuberculosis of every other part of the body, of course, including the lungs, rickets, many skin diseases, varicose ulcers of the longest standing, wounds of war, non-healing operative wounds, osteomyelitis, bed-sores and so on. How shall we proceed ?

In London, in 1921, Dr. Calmette, the illustrious bacteriologist, discussed the tuberculosis question at the International Congress. Elsewhere I have described the " new weapon against tuberculosis " which we may owe to him. He has been able, on the traditional lines of the Pasteur Institute which he adorns, to immunise certain of the lower animals against tuberculous infection by means of an experimental vaccination with modified tuberculous bacilli or their products. But cheap rodents are too far away from us, zoologically, for the most significant experimental results, and there is need for great extension of the work upon anthropoid apes, which are scarce and expensive animals. Dr. Calmette hopes, therefore, to raise enough funds, by international subscription or otherwise, for the acquirement of land, perhaps in some French part of Africa, and of apes enough for the prosecution of his studies ; and some day we may hope, perhaps, to have a " vaccine "—though cows will have nothing to do with it, and one is tempted to suggest that sheep suggest the cerebral affinities of the matter more closely—with which our urban babies throughout the world can be inoculated, so that thereafter, if all goes well, and the process is often enough repeated, they may be able to resist tuberculosis.

I am an avowed believer in Pasteur and modern bacteriology, in vaccination against small-pox, in so-called vaccination against typhoid (which owes so much to Dr. Calmette), in the anti-toxin treatment of diphtheria, and so forth ; and I have tried to direct public attention favourably to the new enterprise of the distinguished French investigator—but, in the light of Leysin, I ask myself whether the medical profession and the public, myself included, have not parted with our senses if we really suppose that this kind of thing is the answer to Dr. Rollier's question, *Comment lutter contre la tuberculose ?* [1]

---

[1] In the two years that have passed since this chapter was first written two new developments in the treatment of tuberculosis have claimed attention, whilst little more has been heard of Dr. Calmette's method. In Geneva, M. Spahlinger has devised a curative serum : in Oxford, Dr. Georges Dreyer, Professor of Pathology, has treated tubercle bacilli with formalin and acetone, removing their fat and then obtaining a new " vaccine," to which he has given the name of " defatted antigen," or " diaplyte." We must wish all success to these efforts. Amongst the crowded and enthusiastic audience at Dr. Dreyer's lecture at St. Mary's Hospital in June, 1923, was one student who had spent the past four years in studying and

No, indeed. Cannot we see the sun at high noon ? Have we learnt nothing, in Great Britain, from the twelve years' record of our national sanatoria for consumption, only fourteen cases in a thousand of the industrial patients visiting which can be recorded as cured ? Let us rub our eyes, and begin to look freshly about us, as if we were intelligent children approaching the matter for the first time.

We shall have to think for ourselves. The light of day was not upon the programme of the 1921 International Conference Against Tuberculosis in London, and it was never mentioned. The Conference, a pitifully disappointing affair, principally assured us, through Dr. Calmette, that latent tuberculosis infectivity is so widespread as to discount our hopes of stopping infection by confining advanced cases in sanatoria. This is very cheerful news, indeed ! When the Conference meets in Washington in 1924, will Americans have heard of the sun ? I leave this question as I asked it in 1921— my American publishers supply the answer herewith.

Clearly our sociology is all wrong. The shameful death rates, especially during the winter, from our

---

recommending the curative and preventive action of sunlight, and even of artificial light, upon tuberculosis, as now practised with magnificent success in a few places in Denmark, Switzerland, France, Italy, Norway, Spain, North America, and Great Britain. It was a duty and a pleasure to go to learn at first hand from Professor Dreyer what can be achieved or hoped from the method of bacteriotherapy in the cure of this disease, and particularly to learn that, in the last analysis, even this extremely artificial and circuitous way of dealing with a disease which should long ago have been abolished depends upon the *vis medicatrix naturæ*. All success indeed to " defatted antigens," especially in their application to diseases which we cannot yet prevent ; but as for tuberculosis, in my view the last word is the first : " In the beginning, God said, ' Let there be light.' "

diseases of darkness, the general lowering of vitality and *joie de vivre*, the gloomy scenes and the uniform sombre colour of the clothes in the streets—all these things lead to a regular hibernal escape from our cities on the part of all who can effect it. The rich or well-to-do go to the Riviera or to Switzerland. On the azure coast they idle, gamble, flirt or what not—but are in the light of day ; in the mountains they skate and ski—and are in the light of day : the better for them. Invalids and delicate children go to Bournemouth, or to convalescent homes at the seaside or in the country. All who can, escape. In the upshot, the results are deplorable, for the overwhelming majority of the population cannot escape. We have some 10,000 deaths every year in Great Britain from so-called " surgical tuberculosis " alone. These resorts and expedients for the few, the rich or a handful of the poor already stricken, are not how to fight against tuberculosis. We are all wrong from the beginning.

First, the whole series of Dr. Rollier's works should be translated into English. The English translations must be put upon the American market. The best and quickest results, in the English-speaking world, will doubtless be obtained in the United States and Canada, partly because of the physical, and partly because of the psychological climate in those countries.

Whilst the laboratory workers elucidate the biology of light, clinicians and philanthropists should avail themselves of, in especial, the superb sun of California, which, unlike that of Leysin, really can be counted upon. If we believe that altitude is an advantage, there are hills to be found there. Possibly the advantages of Canada may be greater. In or near such a spot as Banff, for instance, in the Canadian Rockies, all the advantages of Leysin and more could be reproduced on any scale, and probably the Canadian Pacific Railway would offer no objections. My own observations in Canada, and what I saw at Leysin, lead me to believe that we should find a friend in the cold or cool air. It stimulates. The nervous system, the muscles, the processes of metabolism respond to it. Light and cold seem to be the ideal combination. Perhaps the real merit of altitude resides not in the higher proportion of ultra-violet rays, but in the coolness of air combined with the light. It is impossible to believe that unused muscles could be found so firm and efficient as supports of the skeleton, on the Riviera, for instance, bathed in warm air, as at Leysin. If these views be sound, Canadians should be especially interested, as I suggest in the next chapter.

Readers in the United States have also lessons to learn. In a country so large and wealthy and progressive, tuberculosis should be already unknown, especially after the evidence from New York. Chicago still burns soft coal and is an abominably dirty city. The tuberculosis death rate has been much reduced in recent years by the policy of segregating the infectious, and especially of removing children from infected homes, on the lines of the Œuvre Grancher in Paris. This I learnt, in 1921, from Dr. J. D.

Robertson, Health Commissioner of the City. But there is still much tuberculosis, and there should be none. Philadelphia, the third largest city in the United States, also burns soft coal, and is hatefully dark and dirty. One lesson of the little Republic of Switzerland to the big one in North America is that Chicago and Philadelphia, for instance, ought forthwith to follow the splendid example of New York.

The great surgical "show" of North America, by general consent, is the world-famous clinic of the Mayo Brothers, at Rochester, Minnesota, with its marvellous equipment and organisation. All surgeons from Europe crossing the Atlantic go to Rochester. I suggest to North American surgeons that the greatest surgical "show" in Europe is at Leysin, where surgery has been abolished. The knife is not the weapon wherewith "*lutter contre la tuberculose.*"

Now for Britain. As for the clinical lessons, they are for clinicians. The records, with skiagrams and all, are at their disposal. But the hygienic and sociological lessons are for every reader. The summer goes, and with it the alteration of the clock, which is designed to save daylight. But it is during the winter that the light of the sun is scarcest and most needed. I am satisfied, on the evidence of Canada and Switzerland, that not the very slight cold but the extreme darkness of our urban winters is their fatal factor. We must save sunlight in winter, and this is to be done by the substitution of gas, coke, anthracite, electricity for the burning of soft coal in our cities. My reiterated pleas of twenty years are incalculably reinforced by the lessons of Leysin.

Generally speaking, ill people should not be treated in our cities until this reform is instituted. Hospitals in our present cities are an offence against elementary biology and hygiene. The convenience of consultants who attend the Brompton Hospital for Consumptives or the Great Ormond Street Hospital for Sick Children is a secondary consideration. If most of these patients were treated in the country, in pure air and by heliotherapy, they would get along very well with quite notably few visits from the most illustrious clinicians. (What does any clinician do, at the most, for a patient with tuberculosis or pneumonia ?)

With the rarest exceptions, each of which would be a scandal, reflecting on the past history of the case, operative surgery for tuberculosis should be abandoned. The customary proceeding of opening the lesion, thus making an entry for secondary infection thereafter, is an indefensible barbarism in the light of Leysin. Even the elegant and complete removal of infected cervical glands is the removal of the body's natural and precious outposts against infection.

The laws against the destruction of daylight by coal-smoke and other noxious substances must be amended and strengthened. The public neglect of the Interim Report of Lord Newton's Committee on this subject was pitiful. When I gave evidence again before the Committee in 1921, Lord Newton asked me whether I had heard of any one beside

myself who had read that Report, and I had to
answer " No."   *Quem Deus vult——— !*

A number of distinguished architects wrote to
The Times during the coal strike in 1921 commenting
on the destruction of buildings by coal-smoke, and
hoping that we might learn the lesson taught us by
the clearness and cleanness of the air during the strike.
It is now for architects to recognise their immense
responsibility for houses not made with hands.
According as they do or do not become modern sun-
worshippers in the designing of our new suburbs and
cities and in the construction of houses and buildings,
first, so as to receive the most sunlight, and second,
so as to be inhabitable without the production of coal-
smoke, so will the standard of national health and
vitality rise or fall.   In the fine volume, " London
of the Future," published by Mr. Fisher Unwin for
the London Society, in 1921, Mr. David Barclay
Niven points out that, smoke having been abolished,
and modern construction being quite capable, *all*
buildings should have roof gardens.   And why not ?
To such British pioneers as Professors Patrick
Geddes, Raymond Unwin and Adshead I particularly
commend the lessons of Leysin.

The open-air school as a device for ill children,
here and there, is inadequately valued.   We must
make our urban air clean, and then plant out our
children in it, at school, in such sunlight as we have,
and with the minimum of clothing.   In the sun and
out of the wind—that is where our school children
should be.   Our present ideas of fine school buildings
are part of the general dementia of our urban

civilisation. I used to tease Canadians who, in every town and city, carried me "around" to show me churches and school buildings and the like as indices to their prosperity. Bricks and mortar that confine and darken and stifle the house of life are part of our modern atheism :

As George Fox rais'd his warning cry, " Is it this pile of brick and mortar—these dead floors, windows, rails—you call the Church ? "

" Why, this is not the Church at all—the Church is living, ever living Souls." (From Walt Whitman's "An Old Man's Thought of School.")

The criterion of all institutions, theories, civilisations, sciences is Man : what kind of men, women and children do they produce ? The principal product of Canada is Canadians. By this test our modern sun-worship is justified. To our men with muck-rakes and bistouries and spirit-levels and life-tables and vaccines I commend the spectacle and worship of the dayspring from on high.

Note.—For its historical and suggestive interest I venture to reprint the following letter, which was published by the *New Statesman* after the first appearance of this chapter in its pages :—

MODERN SUN-WORSHIP.
To the Editor of The New Statesman.

Sir,—The interesting and valuable articles by " Lens," and more especially the recent one on the treatment of tuberculosis by exposure to the rays of the sun, prompt me to enter a plea for the urgent necessity of a complete investigation of the physiological action of light of various qualities on the animal organism. Although there has been a notable amount of work done on the action of ultra-violet light on lower organisms, we need much more knowledge of the complex direct and indirect effects on more highly organised beings, including man. There seems to be no doubt that the treatment of tuberculosis by sunlight has had beneficial results, but it is clear from several facts mentioned by " Lens " that the way in which it acts is still obscure. The practical reason for obtaining knowledge of the nature of this action is that some parts of the method adopted by Dr. Rollier, for example, may prove to be unessential, a matter of some consequence in the extended use of the method. It is difficult to believe that the ultra-violet rays themselves play any important part, since it appears that those patients who react by pigmentation of the surface of the skin, a process which prevents the rays in question from penetrating below the surface, derive most benefit. The growth and tone of the muscles, again, suggests that reflex stimulation through the nervous system may turn out to be one of the most powerful modes of action of sunlight and of fresh air. We want to know also how far the actual amount of energy received by the body is significant. There seems to me to be no doubt that the problems involved are worth much more consideration than they have yet received, and the attention directed to them by " Lens " is of great value at the present time.

Yours, etc.,
W. M. BAYLISS.

October 15th, 1921.

CHAPTER VIII

LIGHT AND COLD : A CANADIAN LESSON

THE following chapter is based upon the observations made during a period of several weeks spent in travelling over 5,500 miles in Canada, and suggests the bearing of Canadian records upon the teaching of our great student in this field, Professor Leonard Hill.

As for the United States, let me repeat that Chicago and Philadelphia, which burn much soft coal in their factories, are conspicuous exceptions to the general rule across the Atlantic. Returning to Chicago at night, after visiting some other city of Illinois, as I have done many times, one gets the same brimstone stench that tells the vagrant Londoner, on his approach to Waterloo or Euston, that this is home. So many thousands of miles away from one's own " home town " this infernal and domestic odour of Chicago is naturally very affecting. When I pointed out the contrast with New York to Dr. John Dill Robertson, the able and energetic Health Commissioner of the city, he replied that the convenient fuel of Chicago is soft coal. To this, however, the rejoinder surely is that New York used to burn soft coal, until, in 1905, *as part of the crusade against consumption* (according to the information personally given to me by Dr. Royal S.

Copeland, until recently its Health Commissioner),
the production of " dense " (not " black ") smoke
was forbidden in the city, the consumption death
rate of which fell by one-half in the period 1905–19.
Philadelphia is a fine old city, of great historic
interest to the visitor from England, but, like Chicago,
it is very dirty, because it burns so much soft coal.
It is somewhat disconcerting to the advocate like
myself, who has been lecturing in public on the
smokeless cleanliness of typical American cities, to
receive by post next morning a full-page advertise-
ment from one of our own papers, wherein Philadelphia describes herself and refers, not without
modest pride, to her " fifty miles of smoke stacks."
Every one of those stacks means a barbaric, dirty
and disease-producing waste of the inherited natural
resources of America.

Now for the Canadian evidence. One is, however,
somewhat uncertain as to the attitude of the public
and even the professional mind towards such
questions. For it is evident that our interest in
them and our action upon any answers to them
will largely depend upon the view that we take of
our national health and physique at this time. A
few years ago, on the basis of figures derived from
the physical examination of recruits, we were
content to have ourselves described, by Mr. Lloyd
George, then Prime Minister, not merely *coram
populo*, but *coram mundo*, as " a C 3 nation." A
brief interval having elapsed, during which the
national *personnel* cannot have altered appreciably,
we are told that we are not a C 3 nation any more,

but "the healthiest nation," the envy and despair, so far as our vital statistics and national health are concerned, of "less happy lands." It is necessary to point out that the facts of a not high, but raised, birth rate, obviously the temporary result of demobilisation and already declining accordingly, and of a low general death rate and infant mortality, both the result of the remarkable suppression of summer infantile diarrhœa, afford us no information whatever as to the health, vigour or physique of our population, nor as to the probable condition of the survivors from amongst any year's infants when they are medically examined, some four years after, as school entrants.

No one who has had the opportunity to compare the contemporary products of British stock on the two sides of the Atlantic, both by personal observation and by examination of medical records, as I have done, can doubt that the truth about our now almost wholly urban population is fairly expressed by calling us a C 3 nation. These facts have not been transformed in a few years merely because a certain group of politicians—each conforming to Shakespeare's definition of their kind as "one that would circumvent God"—desire to cut down expenditure upon health and education, or to discredit the projects of the Ministry of Health.

My present contention is that the chief injury done to our lives and health in Britain is inflicted during the winter. "Summer complaints" at all ages we have brought, or are rapidly bringing, under control. Alimentary disorders and infections diminish in importance. The quite astonishing history of summer diarrhœa of infants during the present century is typical of the facts. Let us hold our ground thus gained, fighting water pollution, flies, food infection, and so forth, more strenuously than ever ; but let us now concentrate on our evident next task, which is the precise identification and subsequent amelioration of the factor or factors, *whatever they be*, which make our winters so deadly.

The great, now outstanding, causes of death, which we should conquer next, are *urban, hibernal, respiratory*. Without here making any more than passing reference to pneumonia and bronchitis among adults, I may merely note that, during the past twelve years (ever since the hot, dry, diarrhœal summer of 1911) the highest point of the annual curve of infant mortality has been during no longer the third, but the first trimester ; and, further, that our efforts for infant welfare have accomplished nothing worth mentioning against the mortality during those months, whilst they have been most gloriously successful against the mortality during the summer. It being granted, then, that our winters are deadly, we must next identify the factor or factors which make them so.

At the first blush, the need for any such inquiry is not apparent—perhaps even to the professional observer. The great fact of the winter surely is that it is cold ; what more do we need to ask ? The clinicians and physiologists of, say, 1860, would have inquired no further. But however content the public may be to assume that the cold of winter is our enemy, we cannot do so in the light of certain facts which are familiar to us. In these times sand-bags have gone from window-sills for ever ; we know that it is not the exposed " cabby " but the confined clerk who dies of consumption ; and those of us who, unlike myself, are engaged in clinical practice send our consumptive patients out of heated, confined apartments into air at even quite low temperatures, not concerned about the cold if only the sun be shining.

Further, we have in our time a distinguished physiological observer, already referred to, Professor Leonard Hill, the highest living authority on the relations of the human body to the atmospheric and radiant conditions of its environment, whose long series of researches, published in recent years by the Medical Research Council,[1] are in entire agree-ment with the changed views and practice of clinicians, and have made a new epoch in this fundamental department of physiology. If space availed, one would like to devote a whole section of this chapter to an almost philosophical issue which arises out of his work—as to the question, " Is it possible to have too good a time ? " or, " Are the easiest conditions for mankind the best ? " Physiology, in this regard, and the statistics of cancer, appear to offer the same reply as the History of Successful Nations (one and all defunct) and as religion in its didactic mood everywhere.

[1] See especially " The Science of Ventilation and Open-Air Treat-ment," Part I. (Special Report No. 32, price 10s.) and Part II. (Special Report No. 52, price 6s.) : H.M. Stationery Office, Kingsway, W.C.

On the strictly physiological plane, Leonard Hill's teaching is to the effect that, whilst warmth may be agreeable, it may very easily be devitalising ; that whilst cold may injure under certain conditions, it may be of high value under other conditions ; or, as he puts it in his own words, which we all should do well to memorise and spread everywhere :—

**"Cold is an enemy of the semi-starved,
It is a stimulating friend of the well-fed."**

That is the last sentence of a masterly article which is contributed by our authority to the *International Journal of Public Health* (Vol. II., No. 3, May–June, 1921 ; published by the League of Red Cross Societies, Geneva) under the title "The Relation of Health to Atmospheric Environment." The article is a model of clear, cogent and fascinating exposition, and I greatly regret that so few readers can be expected for it. As I look over it, I naturally want to quote long paragraphs wholesale, in order to convince the present reader, who may not have followed Hill's work nor have realised its immense public importance. At any rate, the logical conclusion of the whole matter is in the sentence above quoted, if we add the words "and well-sunlit."

I went on my third visit to Canada, very much more extended and instructive than its predecessors, with my mind very full of these ideas : that Canada is a great country, but has a cruel winter ; that therefore the population does not increase and cannot be expected to increase, as every believer in the British Empire, and as all loyal Canadians in especial, must desire ; and that the perpetual loss of Canadians to the cosy and comfortable American cities further south is inevitable and must be accepted.

Now for a closer rendering of the facts and their real meaning. In the first place, there is no doubt at all about the cold of the Canadian winter. Of course, Canada is a big place, with varying conditions ; but if we form a picture of the snow falling early in November, and the ground never seen again for five months, whilst the thermometer is around the Fahrenheit zero, and occasionally may go forty degrees lower, we shall not be far wrong. Obviously, therefore, if cold is in question, we really have no cold here, nor any idea of the meaning of the word, as compared with our Canadian cousins. " How do you bear it ? " one naturally asks. The answer is that they bear it very well. For instance, one is shown the ski-jump at Banff, which only allows the brave and skilful devotee a mere 175 feet in the air, 225 being the record, and which is therefore about to be enlarged. The whole story of winter sports is fascinating, not least to the physiologist. By all accounts the Canadians have a very good time during their very cold winter ; and incidentally one learns that *the sun is shining*.

This certainly throws a flood of light upon the matter. For these well-fed Canadians, and their superb children not least, are, taken as a whole, the finest people I have yet seen anywhere in the world. They are very largely Scottish ; very largely indeed, for they have the stature and physique of the old-time rural Scot whom the anthropologists reckoned to be the largest of known men, and who is now about as common in Scotland as the mammoth and the dodo. It is quite a revelation to travel through Ontario, Manitoba, Saskatchewan and Alberta, meeting everywhere a new type of Scot who does not believe in whisky, who has several, or perhaps all, of his own teeth in his head, and whose children are not rickety. They are the most glorious examples of that great race, and the Dominion they have created is, I believe, the hope of the British Empire. The contrast between them and the typical contemporary Scot, as produced in the slums of Edinburgh, Glasgow, or Dundee, is the most poignant demographic fact I have ever seen, and should be proclaimed from the housetops wherever the Union Jack flies.

Many factors are at work to explain this contrast, with all its Imperial implications, hopes and warnings ; but certainly no one who has seen the children of English-speaking *urban* Canada (I am not referring to the rural population, which I scarcely saw) can ever again believe that it is the (practically non-existent) " cold " of our English winters that destroys our children and ourselves. No ; it must be anything but that.

The problem has its ramifications, of course, but I have no doubt that the factor we must incriminate is not the " cold " but the *darkness* of our winters. The cold and the sun of Canada, playing upon the well-fed, produce a splendour of physique, a low rate of disease, an abundant energy of mind, a *joie de vivre*, or national *euphoria*, which must rejoice every amateur of mankind, such as I reckon myself to be. And the lesson for ourselves, the whole matter having been elucidated by our own physiological master, is as clear as day.

We cannot transform our natural climate; but we can and must utterly transform the abominable artificial climate for which we are ourselves responsible in our cities. It is the ironic fact that, having relatively little sunlight here, we value it little; having an abundance in Canada, Canadians value it much. In Winnipeg, as any one may find for himself by consulting the annual reports of Dr. Douglas, its Health Officer, to whom I am much indebted for a most valuable hour spent in his office, more care is taken to prevent the pollution of the atmosphere and to preserve the blessed light of day than in any of the dark, dirty, disease-ridden, heaven-blackening cities of our country. (And I had thought that when I went to Winnipeg I was leaving civilisation, and had actually written home about going to the " wilds of Canada.") Here we receive from the sky not one wavelet of sunlight too many; all are precious and needed. It is a crime against our country to obscure them. Most of our complaints against our climate are unwarranted, if it is heaven we blame; the fault for the urban darkness which is the deadly factor of our winters is our own. It does not suffice that the rich and idle should escape to the Riviera and its sun whilst the great mass of the people who have to produce our wealth in peace and man our trenches in war are exposed, they and their children, to the darkness which can be smelt, falling victims accordingly to the diseases of darkness. We must make our cities really habitable during the winter, as at present they are not. Here is Leonard Hill's teaching (*loc. cit.* p. 240) :—

In England belief in the open, or gas fire, as a source of radiant warmth is justified. The moist, misty, mild weather is thus counteracted. Gas fires must replace coal fires to secure economy of coal energy and remove the pall of smoke, dirt and destruction of vegetable life from the towns, and the great loss of health and wealth these entail. The theory that chemical purity of the air is the one important thing has permitted the establishment of slum cities, undergound places of business, office rooms lit by wells, etc. It must be realised that the carbonic acid is never increased or the oxygen reduced so as to harm to the least extent the occupants. Moreover, after exhaustive experiment by physiologists proof is not forthcoming of those subtle organic poisons supposed to be exhaled by human beings. Massive saliva spray infection from carriers of pathogenic germs and the physical state of the atmosphere depressing the vitality, these are the agents which cause ill health.

Observe that the lessons which Canada has to teach us do not include, on physiological principles, a demand that we should copy Canadian domestic architecture in respect of central heating. Both in Canada and the United States, judicious observers are recognising that the moist, lazy, interior warmth produced in stagnant air by the customary North American practice of central heating is enervating and vicious. But in any case our relatively very mild winters do not involve us in any such problem of domestic heating as the Canadians certainly have. Our climatic conditions make possible and entirely adequate the form of heating which Hill recommends and which alone meets all the indications of physiological science, as well as those of chemistry and physics in respect of the proper use of our soft coal by distilling instead of barbarously burning it. I am still in hopes that, here and there at least, especially under the influence of the final report of Lord Newton's Committee, health and housing committees of local authorities—despite the pusillanimity of the Ministry of Health, which has actually ignored the domestic chimney in its new Bill—and private builders as well, may build our new houses aright from the first, so that we may begin to practise an intelligent modern form of that sunworship which is among the most ancient and surely not the least rational of religions.

CHAPTER IX

THE END OF RICKETS

NEVER again should a case of rickets occur anywhere. It is time to make an end of the "English disease," which can certainly be prevented, or cured, without money and without price, by means of a preventive, or a medicine, which is everywhere available, which is nobody's patent or monopoly, which no doctor is needed to prescribe, nor chemist to dispense, nor parent, nor ratepayer, nor cheerful giver to pay for.

In 1650, the great English anatomist, Francis Glisson, described "the rickets" in one of the masterpieces of medical literature. It has been studied, especially in his country, ever since. An historical survey, of high value and interest, is contributed by a distinguished Scottish student, Dr. Leonard Findlay, to the valuable document [1] of 1918, one of many on this subject which we owe to the Medical Research Council. In that survey Dr. Findlay discussed the "Geographical Distribution" (pp. 15–17) of the disease, and noted many interesting facts thereanent. The group of workers in Glasgow have been known as the Glasgow school,

[1] "A Study of Social and Economic Factors in the Causation of Rickets" (Special Report Series No. 20): H.M. Stationery Office, Kingsway, W.C.

who stand for " social and economic factors " of rickets as against, or in addition to, dietetic factors as such. These latter factors have been specially studied, under the Medical Research Council, by Dr. and Mrs. E. H. Mellanby.[1]

Incomparably most important of all, however, is a fact and a factor which both the Glasgow and the London " schools " missed, and the thing begins to look like material for irony when we find that the really capital discovery was made and duly published in a leading medical journal by an Englishman a generation ago. Sir Ronald Ross has lately commented upon the difficulties involved in the multiplication of medical and scientific " literature." As he says, " No one knows what is known." Really adequate bibliographic methods are required, and their evolution and use must become a special department of scientific work. In this country we are far behind the Germans and the Americans in the kind of organised and concerted effort which is required. Otherwise, in his various references to the geographical distribution of rickets, Dr. Findlay would not have missed the paper which contained the key to the whole problem. But the American students have so advanced their bibliographic methods that a reader like myself, who is prepared to learn in any language or from any source that is intelligible to him, can speedily " discover," as a rule, what has already been discovered on any subject whatever.

The American writers, then, have drawn attention

[1] See the Special Report No. 38 on " Accessory Food Factors."

to a paper on " The Geographical Distribution and
Aetiology of Rickets," published by Dr. Theobald
A. Palm in the *Practitioner*, in October and November, 1890. Dr. Palm, who took his first degree in
Edinburgh so long ago as 1867, is still in practice at
Aylesford, near Maidstone, and his achievement has
remained totally unknown in his own country until
I recently drew attention to it, after reading a paper
that comes from workers at Yale and Johns Hopkins.
The old saying about a prophet's honour is illustrated
once more, of course. The signal homage offered
to our pioneer by the American workers [1] is fully
deserved, and I cannot use the next few inches of
my space, in 1923, better than in quoting verbatim
the conclusions reached by Dr. Palm in 1890, but
ignored and forgotten until now. These conclusions
cannot be improved upon in any particular to-day,
so far as I can see, and they need no further introduction than the simple statement that their author
found the main factor in the causation of rickets
to be deficient sunlight—the capital fact missed by
every other English student, from Glisson himself
onwards, until Germans and Americans found it
experimentally in the present century, and our
workers, headed by Dr. Chick, confirmed it in Vienna
in 1922. Said Dr. Palm long ago :

In conclusion, as practical results of this inquiry, I would
urge the following :—
1. The establishment of means for having systematic and
exact records of the sunshine in the heart of our great cities
as well as at favourite health resorts. A sunshine recorder
at an observatory on some hilltop near a large city is no

[1] *Journal of the American Medical Association*, January 21st, 1922.

guide to the amount of sunshine that reaches the streets and alleys of smoky cities. It is important that the sunshine recorder be of the form which indicates the chemical activity of the sun's rays rather than its heat.

2. The removal of rachitic children as early as possible from large towns to a locality where sunshine abounds and the air is dry and bracing.

3. The establishment of a sanatorium for poor rickety children in some such locality, where the severe development of the disease may be averted and much life and health saved by timely treatment.

4. The systematic use of sun-baths as a preventive and therapeutic measure in rickets and other diseases.

5. That, when a mother has once borne a child which has become rachitic, preventive treatment of the disease in her future children should be adopted, if possible, by change of climate and mode of life in the mother, nothing urged above being inconsistent with the belief that the mother's state of health brought about by the same causes predisposes her offspring to rickets.

6. The education of the public to the appreciation of sunshine as a means of health. Many persons seem to prefer darkness to light in their dwellings out of ignorance, thoughtlessness, or even an economic regard for carpets and curtains. Let people understand that sunshine in the dwelling not only reveals unsuspected dirt, but is Nature's universal disinfectant as well as a stimulant and tonic. Such knowledge will also stimulate efforts for the abatement of smoke and for the multiplication of open spaces, especially as playgrounds for the children of the poor.

Dr. Findlay doubts whether Homer's description of Thersites, or a paragraph in Hippocrates, indicates rickets, and he regards Soranus, who practised in Rome in the second century of our era, as the first writer to describe the disease beyond dispute. In any case, medical men have been studying rickets for a very long time—and in our own country with appallingly abundant and never-failing "clinical material"—but it remained for Dr. Palm in 1890 to discover the principal fact about it. When I

think of all the oceans of " medicine " administered
to infants and children lying in the shade, all the
theories as to causation, all the surgical operations
on knock-knee, all the volumes and monographs and
learned disquisitions on what turns out to be simply
one of the diseases of darkness, I long for the
composite pen of a Rabelais, a Swift, a Samuel
Butler, an Anatole France and a Bernard Shaw to
laugh (or cry) at the blind folly of the seeming
wisest of mankind. For some 2,000 years we have
been staring at rickets, with our backs to the light,
and taxes on windows, and Heaven knows what
conglomeration of stupidities, and have seen no
more than as if the only use we had for glass were
to fit us with eyes.[1]

During the present century many students have
made progress. Buchholz cured rickets by light in
1904 ; Rollier has been curing rickets by light for
many years at Leysin, and photographs of the
typical results are to be found in his " La Cure
de Soleil," 1914 ; Huldschinsky reported in 1919,
attributing special value to the ultra-violet rays ;
he was confirmed by many other observers in
Germany too numerous to mention, and then the
Americans took the matter up in great style and
settled it. A few minutes daily effect a cure in two
to three weeks, after a *total exposure* of, say, four
and a half hours or so.

Meanwhile, the children of Sheffield, under the
darkness which can be smelt, are receiving cod-liver

---

[1] By the way, if the ultra-violet be the saving rays, and if glass
arrests them, we must " think again " as to window panes.

oil for their rickets, whilst Dr. F. E. Wynne, the Professor of Public Health and Medical Officer of Health in that city, publicly describes as a "hasty assumption" my statement that sunlight can cure or prevent rickets. In Sheffield, of all places, whilst Essen is smokeless and sunny, official efforts are made, in the name of public health, to throw doubt upon the virtues of the sunlight. Again I covet that composite pen of all the master ironists of all ages ! But, failing it, I commend Dr. Palm's recommendations to the citizens of Sheffield.

Not one word against cod-liver oil do I suggest. Until the shame of Sheffield's smoke is ended, or until such sunlight as Sheffield has is used for childhood, as Dr. Palm suggested, let cod-liver oil be bought and given to the children. The vitamin in it was probably made by sunlight falling on the green plankton in the far waters of the North Atlantic, and thence, *viâ* other creatures, reached the cod, and the cod's liver, whence at length it gets into the blood of Sheffield children. But why not use the sun, even in Sheffield, directly ?

Any neglect of the dietary factors of rickets, to which I have been directing public attention ever since the earlier work of Professor E. H. Mellanby, is here repudiated. The student will necessarily study the authoritative new statement [1] on the subject which we owe to the Medical Research Council, and in which the dietary factors are given

[1] "Studies of Rickets in Vienna, 1919–22" (Report to the Accessory Food Factors Committee appointed jointly by the Medical Research Council and the Lister Institute), 1923; H.M. Stationery Office, Kingsway, W.C. (7s. 6d. net.)

at least their full measure of importance. On the climatic aspect one more note.

The great record of tropical medicine in the present century illustrates the importance of the distribution of disease. If an " intermediate host " be essential, like the *Anopheles* mosquito in malaria, or the *Stegomyia* mosquito in yellow fever, then evidently the geographical facts of those insects are of the first importance. And, when such problems are still to be solved, the key might be found if, for instance, a properly made survey showed that the distribution of the disease coincided with that of some insect which had never hitherto been thought of in that relation. An admirable volume on " The Geography of Disease," [1] by the late Dr. F. G. Clemow, was published just twenty years ago, and has ever since been valued on my shelves. A very fair indication of the quality of the author may be gained from the fact that, though he was unaware of the paper published by Dr. T. A. Palm in the *Practitioner* in 1890, he writes of rickets that " the infrequency of the disease in warm countries . . . is largely due to the beneficent influence on young children of sunlight and fresh air." The section of his work dealing with cancer is of very great interest, and should long ago have led to more active inquiry by the geographical and statistical method.

In the magnificent volume on the distribution of cancer mortality throughout the world, published by the Prudential Insurance Company of America,

[1] In the Cambridge Geographical Series: Cambridge University Press, 1903.

and compiled by their masterly statistician, Dr. Frederick L. Hoffman, one has naturally sought for any evidence as to any possible relation between the light factor and cancer—none the less because of the known power of certain of the Röntgen rays to produce cutaneous cancer, and of certain others to kill malignant cells, and of intense tropical or subtropical sunlight, after a long time, to produce cancer of the skin, as especially studied in Queensland. No such correlation appears likely to me from the existing data: Scotland, Switzerland, Maine and California, for instance, differ extremely in respect of the light factor of climate, and all have very high cancer death rates.

CHAPTER X

SUNLIGHT AND TUBERCULOSIS

INCOMPARABLY the best way to treat a patient suffering from rickets or tuberculosis, or any of the other diseases of darkness, is by heliotherapy. The ill person, blanched and devitalised by light-starvation, and the specific disease which has now complicated it, is gradually, slowly, cautiously restored to the light for lack of which he is dying. His unaccustomed skin must be exposed, during five minutes, thrice, at intervals, for the feet alone, during the first day, to direct sunlight. Even so much will very likely cause tenderness and swelling, signs of reaction, in a group of tuberculous glands in the neck, far away from the exposed feet. On the second day the feet may be uncovered thrice for ten minutes, and so, by slow degrees, the skin may be accustomed to the light until, after a fortnight, the patient may be completely exposed from the beginning, and remain so perhaps for three or four hours. The skin will become gradually pigmented, and with the pigmentation will come an improvement in the patient's condition, the two being closely but obscurely correlated. No drugs need or should be given, nor is cod-liver oil needed, wonderful drug though it be. The sunlight does all, given that the patient has air to breathe, simple food to eat, and water to drink. Current medical and surgical methods in the treatment of these diseases are seen to be pure foolishness or cruelty, or both, in the light of heliotherapy.

I here repeat the most explicit and conspicuous warning against the idea that any uninstructed person can practise heliotherapy by rule of thumb without grave danger. The most tragic accidents have occurred, and there will be many more. The curative agent is the light, and not the heat, of the sun. In varying proportions, they reach us together ; but the light stimulates, whilst the heat enervates. There have been those who, never having seen heliotherapy in practice, nor having read a line by any of its students, have begun by exposing the chests of patients suffering from pulmonary tuberculosis to the midday sun, and have then concluded from the consequent fever, spitting of blood, and early end of the case that sunlight is useless in pulmonary tuberculosis. I totally repudiate responsibility for any accident or disagreeable event, great or small, that may follow attempts at heliotherapy without sense, caution, and study. The whole thing depends upon the healing power of nature ; it is a vital reaction on the part of the patient's body to certain modes of stimulation and nutrition available in the sun's rays. It therefore partakes of the subtlety, variety, and spontaneity of life ; each case is to be regarded as personal and unique, and all statements about times and seasons and dosages are to be regarded as mere average indications of the kind of thing that would apply in many instances. I do not practise medicine; I have no solarium for any one outside my own household; I do not know the names of any private practitioners, among all the tens of thousands in this country, who practise heliotherapy, or who can even be named as authorities upon it. I am overwhelmed with letters and inquiries on this matter from the lay public and the medical profession, and the only answer I now can make is to point to Dr. Rollier's book.

His address is Leysin, Switzerland, and the way to write to him is to write to him, as I am weary of telling inquirers. I have no desire to get people to write to him or to send patients to him. The meaning of his work is that only owing to our folly and ignorance has he any work to do. When the civilised world understands what his work means, the diseases of darkness will vanish, and he will have no patients to treat—the consummation devoutly to be wished, for which I work. Meanwhile, the capital fact is that, wherever the principles of heliotherapy are understood its results can be obtained. The beauty of this business is that it is no one's patent, and needs no chemist to dispense, nor protected manufacturers to prepare. The handful of clinicians who have discovered the sun may each incline to think that his special combination of circumstances furnishes the unique requirement, but there is nothing in that. In our own country, at the Treloar Hospital, Sir Henry Gauvain has been obtaining results like Rollier's at Alton and Hayling Island; Dr. Gordon Pugh gets them at Queen Mary's Hospital for Children at Carshalton; they are on the way to being obtained at the Heritage Craft Schools at Chailey, in Sussex; they are obtained at the J. N. Adam Memorial Hospital, at Perrysburg, in the United States; at the Villa Santa Maria, outside Cannes; at the Istituto Elioterapico, outside San Remo; in Spain, near Barcelona; and in Norway, in and outside Christiania. The common fact in all these places, nearly all of which I have visited during the inquiry of the last few years, is that they employ the sun. Wherever the sun shines, any one who will use patience and respect and intelligence can obtain similar results. The evidence I saw in the confined urban atmosphere of Columbia University, New York, last December, and the latest evidence from Copenhagen and the London Hospital, make that clear.

Thanks to the recent awakening on the subject, the authorities at the "London" began, in August, 1922, as we have seen elsewhere, to expose some of their patients to the "general light bath," quite apart from any local irradiation of diseased areas. In brief, many cases which could not be cured by the local action of light have been cured by the general light bath without exposure of the diseased area to the light at all. The cure rate has risen from about 65 to about 95 per cent. Seeing that Rollier began in 1903, 1922 seems rather late for this development, so simple and easy and inexpensive and lovely in result, on the part of an institution which was actually using light three years before Rollier began; but that is the way in which things happen in our country, and the "London" still remains the pioneer. What are the other hospitals going to do, and when ? And who will be the first private practitioner, the first children's doctor, the first infants' specialist, to apply the new discoveries ? For the first time since I " qualified " to practise medicine I almost wish I did so !

Every one will be practising heliotherapy soon, and Rollier's must be their text-book. It is comprehensive, including a masterly discussion of the " scientific basis of heliotherapy," by Dr. Rosselet, a chapter on the use of the X-rays for diagnosis by Dr. Schmid, one on the heliotherapy of non-tuberculous diseases by Dr. Amstad, and so forth. Very formidable vested interests in the knife and the bottle will have to be combated, but they will assuredly yield to the facts recorded in this volume, and to the practice to which it constitutes the first complete and authoritative guide in our language.

So much for ill people and for the colossal host of those whose profession it is to treat ill people. My own concern is not with heliotherapy at all, except as the evidence upon which we must state the case for heliohygiene.

The real meaning of heliotherapy is that we should restore to our urban lives the sunlight by which all life is maintained, and that therefore we should abolish the plague cloud of coal-smoke which deprives us, during the winters, of more than half our sunlight—and especially of those lower notes in the ultra-violet which are probably the most valuable of all that the sun sends us. An admirable series of practical recommendations has been unanimously made by the authoritative and representative committee which recently studied the subject under the chairmanship of Lord Newton. The Ministry of Health has introduced a Bill which, in its present form, is a monument of pusillanimity and futility as regards the industrial and the domestic chimney alike. Much could and should be done to deal with the industrial chimney, and the Minister of Health has a unique opportunity, in connection with the country's new houses, to equip them so that they shall conform to what Mr. E. D. Simon, in his admirable little volume of 1922, called " The Smokeless City." [1]

But as for the domestic chimney, we can only say that houses are being built to make smoke, as ever, despite the recommendations of the Ministry of Health's own Committee; whilst the Federation of British Industries has protested against any legislation as being liable to ruin the industries of our country. We have yet to learn from these manufacturers, in Sheffield and elsewhere, why Essen should be smokeless while Sheffield turns day into worse than night. My own view is the hackneyed but everlasting truth :

> " Ill fares the land, to hastening ills a prey,
> Where wealth accumulates and men decay."

[1] " The Smokeless City," by E. D. Simon, Lord Mayor of Manchester, and Marion Fitzgerald, with an Introduction by Lord Newton: Longmans Green. (1s. 6d.)

CHAPTER XI

SUNLIGHT AND BOVINE TUBERCULOSIS

EVER since the discovery of the tubercle bacillus in 1881, we have been hypnotised by our one-eyed staring at it through the microscope, and have called it *the* cause of tuberculosis without remembering that no infection can occur without susceptibility, and that the capacity to be infected is as much a necessary factor of tuberculosis or any other infection as is the infective agent itself. The evidence of the war and the after-war in Vienna and elsewhere has recently caused medical opinion everywhere to open both eyes, forget the tubercle bacillus for a moment, and look around at the conditions of nutrition, or malnutrition, which cause us either to be consumers of the tubercle bacillus, if it enters us, or to be consumed by it. A new era in the study of nutrition dates from the German and American experiments on sunlight, and begins to explain, or to construct a key for the explanation of, the incomparable success of sunlight against tuberculosis.

But, of course, we must not ignore infection, nor propose to dismiss bacteriology merely because we have reminded ourselves of nutrition. Thus, in a later chapter it is sought to show that by pasteurisation of our milk supply we may hope to reduce the amount of tuberculous (and other) infection. We accept as a constant factor, so to say, the presence of tuberculosis in our dairy cattle, and seek to protect ourselves by killing the bacilli in their milk.

We may go farther and seek to eliminate infection by tests for tuberculosis and by the slaughter of tuberculous cows, or by the "vaccination," now being attempted, of calves with Dr. Dreyer's "Diaplyte." As every one knows, this is a matter of difficulty, expense, and controversy.

But here we may go farther still, reiterating, with a new argument, a favourite theme. If it be true that tuberculosis in ourselves is a disease due to malnutrition and lowered resistance to infection, and that good nutrition, dependent on sunlight, open air, and enough fresh food, causes us to bear a charmed life amidst perpetual attacks by the infective agent—ought not similar principles to apply to our cattle ? Surely tuberculosis must be a disease of darkness amongst them as amongst us ; and surely a more excellent way than to pasteurise our milk, or to detect and kill tuberculous cattle, would be to apply the principles of hygiene and good nutrition to them as to ourselves.

Tuberculosis is being not only studied and fought, but rapidly conquered in North America. The results of inquiry along a certain line have just been published by Dr. J. A. Kiernan, of the United States Department of Agriculture, and they amount to this : that in North America tuberculosis afflicts cattle just in proportion to the degree in which they live in the dark and under cover. The stabling of cattle is the danger to them. "Range cattle" are almost free from the disease. Where cattle are crowded, stabled, darkened, as in New York State, there may be 26 per cent. or more of tuberculosis amongst them, whereas "in the north-western States of the Union, where the winters are severe, few areas have more than 3 per cent. tuberculous cattle." This continent-wide survey of the facts is in strict conformity with everything that we are coming to learn and teach about tuberculosis in mankind ; and it is in precise agreement with the physiological researches of our own great student, Professor Leonard Hill, F.R.S., Director of the Department of Applied Physiology under the Medical Research Council. It is also in conformity with the answer returned to me when on a visit of study to Switzerland some time ago. I expressed astonishment that tuberculosis should exist among cattle in a country so favoured with sunlight, air, and fresh food : " But," my medical informant replied, " our farmers shut their cattle in the dark deliberately believing that thus their milk is improved."

It is my hope that veterinary students will follow up this matter from their standpoint, and that Professor Leonard Hill may think it worth while to extend his observations to cattle in view of this North American evidence.

But let us not suppose that there is anything really new in all this. Far from it. Nothing is more remarkable than the fashion in which genius, which Carlyle defined as " the clearer presence of God Most High in a man," anticipates the laboured steps of science. In 1906 I defined alcohol as a "racial poison," and have ever since sought to protect our young parents, and especially our expectant mothers from it; but inquiry into the history of this idea led me back to Judges, Chapter XIII., where the "Angel of the Lord," we are told, gave precise ante-natal instructions and warnings against wine and strong drink to her whose task it should be to mother a hero. And, in this matter of tuberculosis among cattle, no man of science has any claims to priority, for it was Honoré de Balzac, in his lovely tale, "The Country Doctor," who puts into the mouth of that magnificent character just such directions for the hygiene of cattle according to Nature's laws as we now see to be indicated in virtue of continent-wide statistical comparison of tuberculin tests. If any student of Balzac knows how, if not by the sheer insight of genius, Balzac acquired the veterinary and vital wisdom which he utters through the mouth of the country doctor, I should be deeply interested in the discovery.

Meanwhile, why should we not adopt light and air for our cattle? Surely all the evidence, of all kinds, is unanimous. We must get back to first principles in and for our lives, and in and for the lives of our domestic animals. "Nature is to be commanded," said Francis Bacon, "only by obeying her."

In a later chapter we shall see that, quite apart from tuberculosis, the actual quality, in certain essential respects, of cow's milk depends in part upon the cow's exposure to or deprivation of sunlight.

CHAPTER XII

THE LESSONS OF A FUR-FOX FARM

PRINCE EDWARD ISLAND, the island-province of Canada, is now reviving, with great success, an industry which was booming before the war, and which is of interest alike to the naturalist, to the humanitarian, and to the eugenist. The trapping of wild animals for their fur is associated with the most hideous cruelty, comparable in many instances with the infamies of egret hunting and the pursuit of other birds for their plumage. But, on this island, some thirty years ago, as I am informed, an illiterate but intelligent man began to breed the silver fox, a very rare creature that occurs as a kind of sport from the ordinary red fox ; and during a visit to the island in 1922, I was taken to a fox ranch, which shows how this industry has developed, and which incidentally illustrates perfectly every principle of eugenics without exception.

Being one of those defenders of vivisection who loathe all cruelty to animals, I had first to be assured that I should see no cruelty ; nor did I. All that has gone. This is a place where a rare and precious wild animal is bred for its pelt ; but the condition of the skin, as any dermatologist will tell you, depends upon the general health, and the general health, as any psychologist or physician will tell you, depends upon happiness, so that nothing is to be won in this competitive industry unless cruelty be left out. The owner of the ranch I saw was a colonel in the Canadian forces during the war, and is not exactly a sentimentalist, but he calls his animals " dear " when he is persuading-pushing them through a passage into the open ; and he kills them with a hypodermic injection over the heart, which obliterates consciousness in a few seconds.

For success, in the first place, you must begin with the very finest animals obtainable. The skin gives them their value, and in judging the living animals, as at the big shows held in Toronto, 85 per cent. of the marks are given for that ; but it is found that there is a high correlation between the state of the pelt and the other points of the animal. Heredity, of course, asserts itself strongly, and the breeders who aim at numbers and do not practise a rigorous selection are very soon outclassed in quality. Only one policy pays in the long run, and that is the most critical and ruthless selection of the best for parenthood. The others may be sold or pelted, but they are not bred from. In making additions to the stock the same principle is followed, whatever the price that must be paid. In thus breeding only from the best, and in excluding all inferior additions, the fur-fox farmer is practising exactly the principles on which I counsel Canadians and others to " encourage worthy parenthood " and to " discourage unworthy parenthood " : positive and negative eugenics respectively, in my terminology.

For the birth of the young, conditions of seclusion

and peace must be preserved. A clever box, containing another box, is placed in communication with the cage, and there, in the dark and quiet, as if in the hollow of a fallen tree, the young may be born. The mother's long, bushy and beautiful tail is curled round the cubs, and at this time the father is very good to her, bringing all the food he obtains, and would surely starve himself for her if necessary. (Cats have succeeded as foster-mothers.) When the foxes are caught and held up by tail and hind legs the visitor can study the fur of the young and the adult and observe its changes, its double character, and the peculiarities of the white or white-ringed hairs which make this fur inimitable and thus determine its exceedingly high cost.

We are plagued in Great Britain with a species of pseudo-eugenist whose only real concern is to reduce expenditure on the young of our country, and who accordingly decries the importance of " nurture " as contrasted with " nature " (to use the terms that my master Galton took from Shakespeare); and we also have the laboratory workers and other theorists who strive to estimate the relative weight of the factors of nurture and nature in the production of any characteristic of a living creature. These workers observe the utmost existing limits of nature in different individuals, whilst observing differences of nurture within very small and arbitrarily-determined limits (for instance, they use a constant atmosphere for inhalation in all cases); then they tell us that nature is so many times more potent than nurture. More sterile and stupid inquiries and argu-

ments than these there never were. It is refreshing
to turn to the practice of men who are not merely
arguing about eugenics, but (though in a relatively
humble species of animal) are successfully practising it.

Of course, they take the utmost interest in nurture,
from the first ante-natal moment of their creatures
until they choose the means wherewith to kill them.
Of course, being practical men with something to
do, they do not argue about nature and nurture, nor
do they discuss the relative importance of the
psychical and physical factors of the latter. They
simply attend to everything. Thus, much care is
taken not to frighten the animals, who are exceedingly timid, and vanish at the approach of even
those they know. Especially when the young are
born is the rule of quiet, the minimum of movement
and disturbance, observed.

After we had withdrawn we saw the animals come
out and peer about and look at us curiously and sniff
the wires which we had touched, and then I realised
that there were many foxes (200 in fact) living
where previously scarce one could be seen. Any
approach towards domestication seems unknown,
or almost so, here, though in our own Zoological
Gardens in London I have seen a tame fox that
wagged its tail like a dog, and was quite as charming.
A former worker on the ranch I saw in Prince Edward
Island became too incautious with the animals and
" quitted " after one of them had firmly secured his
nose between its jaws.

On the physical side there are many problems to

solve. Parasitic infection is one—a kind of hook-worm, which is dosed with carbon tetrachloride ; a kind of distemper ; fleas ; infections of the ear, and so on. A regular bacteriological service has to be maintained. Apart from all that, there are the positive factors of nutrition, and what was my interest and amusement when my host began spontaneously to dilate on two factors which I had not mentioned to him. He had been a chemist, and looks at nutrition biochemically. Above all, he believes in cod-liver oil. He makes a special biscuit, in very large demand on other farms, containing not only linseed meal, and so forth, but a constant quantity of cod-liver oil. I went to see these biscuits made, and was surprised to find them quite palat-able. In Newfoundland, I am told, fox-farming is to develop, with the remains of cod as the principal diet of the animals. The oil used here is not the crudest, but is not highly refined, and doubtless is very rich accordingly in vitamin A. Certainly, I saw nothing like rickets in the movements and form, the jaws and the teeth, of these lovely animals ; and no wonder, when my host, without any prompting from me, began to dilate upon the sunlight which is the great feature of Canada, and the glory and benison of the long and cold Canadian winter. The utmost use is made of the sunlight, he said ; nothing else is found so effective as a disin-fectant of the cages, and, indeed, the sunlight solves that problem. Just like the chamois in Switzerland, the foxes love the sunlight and bask in it during the summer mornings, and then retreat from the midday heat. They thus show their superiority of sense over those jealous critics of the sun-cure in Britain, whom nothing can induce to distinguish between the sun's light and the sun's heat. (*Cf.* " A pleasant thing it is for the eyes to behold the sun " ; and " Fear no more the heat of the sun.") At this point I wished for the company of a few leaders of opinion from my own country, but that, after a fourth visit to North America, one begins to feel that Britain is hopeless. Of course it is not ; but the present difference in educability and in energy is so great that one may almost be forgiven for thinking so.

The exquisite pelts which are the products of such a ranch as I have tried to describe are valued chiefly, I fear, because they are rare and cannot be imitated. Well, worse things have been done to gratify feminine vanity ; and the process in this case illustrates every contention of those who teach that the laws of life are the laws of all life, and that the only way in which to make the world a better place to live in is to make better people to live in the world.

CHAPTER XIII

SUNLIGHT AND MILK

AFTER every visit to Canada and the United States, I return to my native land with increased concern at the apathy and stupor of the public regarding the food of foods.

Milk is nothing less than that. Whatever else we consume was assuredly not designed for us by Nature. The muscles of the sheep were meant to serve the sheep, not to make mutton chops for us ; the grain of the wheat is for the next generation of wheat, and so on. Milk alone, of all that we eat, is evolved and contrived by Nature in order to be a food. As the science of dietetics advances, new valuations need to be set upon this or that article of consumption. Traditional views of, say, beef and beer need to be revised. Milk, like all else, comes under reconsideration, but always with higher marks than we had allotted to it before. The recent discovery and elucidation of vitamins, for instance, which has required us to put another black mark against beer, since that is destitute of them, has added even further to our appreciation of milk. Indeed, a good principle of dietetic research would be to assume, as a working hypothesis, that whatever Nature puts into the only food she has ever made is of dietetic value, and that whatever is not there is of none.

Sound and persistent teaching on the value of milk as the food of foods has had its result in Canada and the States. Wherever one goes, opinion and practice are the same. In Great Britain the people consume about a quarter of a pint per head per day, according to the official estimates accepted by the Astor Committee, which adds, in its report, that " this is less than half the normal average consumption of the city of New York." But since the advent of prohibition in the United States and in the greater part of Canada the consumption of milk has markedly and steadily increased, the latest figure for the United States being ·78 of a pint per head per day, which is *more than three times* as much as we consume in this country.

It is not merely that, as every one knows or should know, the children of English-speaking North America are vastly better fed in this respect than ours. The contrast in consumption depends also upon the high value which is set upon milk by adults. During my first visit, in 1919, when big, broad-shouldered men entered a restaurant, sat down opposite me and ordered glasses of milk, I was repeatedly surprised. Were these burly, hearty fellows ill ? By no means ; they were merely ordering the food which had laid the foundations of their superb physique, and by which they were maintaining it.

The comparative recentness of the full popular appreciation of milk in North America is illustrated by the view, taken during the war, when certain States on the Pacific went " dry," that the Allied cause would be injured by the retardation of shipbuilding in the absence of beer. But statistical observation showed in due course that the milk-drinking Pacific shipbuilders were far outpacing their beer-drinking rivals on the Atlantic seaboard.

It is well known that the Japanese, a wonderful people ambitious for world empire, have been chagrined and concerned for many years at the comparative shortness and lightness of their physique. At one time a systematic attempt was made by them to increase their consumption of meat, for which they have no great liking. But, in view of more recent researches in dietetics, the Japanese have decided that milk, of which they have hitherto consumed extremely little, their country having very few cows, is what I have long called it, the food of foods, and, after due consultation, they are now engaging expert American advice in order greatly to increase their milk supply.

In his famous presidential address to the British Association, now some quarter of a century ago, Sir William Crookes suggested that the superiority of Western over Eastern civilisation really depends upon the superiority of wheat over rice. That lecture, expanded into a volume on "The Wheat Problem" (Longmans, Green & Co.), is and will remain a masterpiece. At my suggestion, the late Lord Rhondda, during the war, generously defrayed the cost of a new edition, the preparation of which was the last piece of work which we owe to its author. But whilst the high place of wheat as a cereal cannot be challenged, I have been wondering, during the last decade, and even before I persuaded my venerable friend to republish his book as a piece of war-work, whether the very marked contrast between the consumption of milk in Europe and in the Far East may not be a more important factor of power than the superiority of wheat to rice. Similarly, in the light of recent dietetics, one is wondering whether, in the combination of porridge and milk which, in past years, made country-bred Scotsmen actually the tallest and biggest of living men—superb in physique and courage and energy— the milk may not have been more important than the cereal. This I have certainly observed, that the superb children and adults of Western Canada in especial—the finest children undoubtedly that I have ever seen in any country in the world hitherto—are fed most abundantly on milk, whilst the use of oatmeal has very greatly declined amongst them, though a very large proportion of them are of Scottish stock.

Other things being equal—and they are not equal, but for the most part are very heavily balanced against us—a Great Britain consuming, say, one-third as much milk per head as the English-speaking people of North America cannot possibly expect to stay the pace with Canada and the States in the race of nations. And the fact that Japan, the recent claimant for a place second to none in the world's affairs, is now greatly increasing her milk supply for the production of the healthy physique upon which all national efficiency depends, should cause us to bethink ourselves in time.

The paradox of milk is that, as we have it for the

most part, it continually distributes not only life and health, but also death and disease to those who consume it. The typical instance of tuberculosis may be cited. More than forty years have passed since the discovery of the tubercle bacillus by Koch in 1881. When I was a medical student in Edinburgh, near the end of the nineteenth century, my surgical teacher, Professor John Chiene, on my first day in his wards, stood at the door and pointed with his finger successively at more than half the patients lying there, uttering the one word "milk" as he indicated each bed. Surgical tuberculosis, as we still wrongly call it, was and is one of the curses of Scotland. It would have swamped the Royal Infirmary of Edinburgh and the Sick Children's Hospital if all the cases that came had been admitted. The extreme and shameful prevalence of this disease in Scotland, as compared with the continent of Europe, or even with England, must be correlated with the facts that in Scotland the supply of sunlight is poor, and pasteurisation was and still is so generally neglected.

In the States and in Canada one is struck by the extreme relative rarity of evidence of surgical tuberculosis in the streets. Inquiry into the statistical facts confirms these impressions. I asked Dr. John Dill Robertson, Health Commissioner of the city of Chicago, why I saw so little evidence of surgical tuberculosis in the streets, and he replied that all the milk consumed in that city is pasteurised. In Winnipeg, a magnificent city of 220,000 inhabitants, I consulted Dr. A. J. Douglas, the Medical Officer of Health. His annual report for 1919 is now before me. During that year the people of Winnipeg drank considerably more than twice as much milk as we do, the figure of 0·56 pint per head per day concerning fresh milk only, and not including condensed milk, cream, milk powder, etc. Nevertheless, the report proceeds :—

"All this, however, does not prove that we have nothing to complain of, or that we should be satisfied. . . . We should not be satisfied with a half pint *per capita* consumption, but should endeavour to make it a three-quarter or even a whole pint."

The greater part of Winnipeg milk is pasteurised. I remarked, as usual in North America, the extreme rarity of evidence of surgical tuberculosis in the streets. (I do not remember having seen a hunchback in North America in four visits of something under three months each.) On turning to the tables of mortal statistics in the report before me I find that, whilst some surgical tuberculosis still exists in Winnipeg, it is becoming negligible. The figures are tiny. Nor need one be surprised, in a sunny city, where people drink an abundance of milk and its products, than which no better sources of resistance to tuberculosis exist, and where the milk that protects them is for the most part prevented from simultaneously infecting them.

Now let us take another type of infection that is conveyed in milk. When I called on Dr. Royal S. Copeland, Health Commissioner for New York City, in September, 1920, I wished to talk to him about New York air, but he wished to talk to me about London milk. Never shall I forget the keen anxiety with which he pulled a copy of the Astor Report out of his desk and turned to p. 77—which I knew only too well—pointing to the examination of twenty-eight samples of milk supplied to mothers attending Infant Welfare Centres in my city, and saying that *only one* of those samples would be allowed to be sold in his. All the rest were so abominably contaminated with *bacillus coli* from the cow's bowel that the sanitary regulations of New York would allow them to be sold only for such purposes as, say, making artificial buttons. They were typical examples of the mixture of milk and muck by which we nourish and poison ourselves in this our mother of nations.

It is an interesting point, and new to me, that according to evidence presented to and accepted by Lord Newton's Committee on Air Pollution, there is a relation between the subject on which I wanted information from Dr. Copeland and that on which, as an admirer and lover of England, he was so solicitous to remind me ; for it has been shown that our milk supply in Great Britain is injured by the action of smoke on the vegetation on which our cows feed. At my public lectures during recent years on the smoke question, the suggestion has sometimes been made that, after all, there is the wind which blows the smoke away. But the smoke has to be paid for nevertheless. If it be removed from the city it spoils the country. My reply to this question is, first, to quote the observed effect of smoke on milk production, and, second, to quote the remarks of flying men to me when lecturing on this subject at the Royal Aircraft Establishment, Farnborough—that, with the wind in the right direction, the airman can see the smoke of the burning of modern Babylon as far as Bournemouth.

The immense consumption of ice cream in Canada and the States by men, women and children of all ages and classes cannot but interest the visitor. He has heard, of course, how deleterious are the products of the ice cream parlour to the digestion. All one can say on this is that, if to eat heartily of all manner of food, including ice cream, with palpable enjoyment, and then to work or play no less heartily and with consummate success in both activities, as is the general rule in the States and Canada—if these be the symptoms of indigestion, then indigestion is good enough for me. The truth doubtless is that the general use of cream and sugar and fruit in this highly *palatable*—and *therefore*, as we know from the classical researches of Pawlow, in Petrograd, highly *digestible*—form must be amongst the factors of that abounding vigour and *joie de vivre* which are the perpetual delight of every lover of his kind in North America. I long for the wide establishment, in our country, of the ideal public-house, of which we talk so much here, without the least idea of what we mean—the places, common in all the small and large towns and cities of Canada and the States, where, amid spotless surroundings, clean-clothed attendants provide individual visitors of any age and either sex, couples, parties, residents, travellers, rich and poor, with pure food and drink and refreshment, usually to the accompaniment of

music at almost all hours, for most moderate cost,
and without a vestige or a possibility of any intoxica-
tion, infection, danger or degradation to those who
are served or those who serve. I remember one
such in a town of 4,000 persons, with tiled walls
and floor, ventilating fans, well-shaded lights, a
gramophone giving us Kreisler's rendering of
Dvorak's "Humoresque," responsible citizens, boys
and girls, all happy together, and then a young
father wheeling in a sleeping baby in its perambu-
lator, with its mother beside him. I am wholly at a
loss to imagine what factor or factors could be added
to improve the title of such a place—one of hundreds
of thousands—to the name of the ideal public-house.
Pasteurised cream and fresh fruit (not syrups) were
its foundations, and the critical reader will observe
that, even if vitamin C be deficient in the former,
it abounds in the latter. A fortune in his pocket
and a peer's coronet on his head should await the
man who would give us these blessings in Britain.

The conclusion of the whole matter is that, if we
are to restore the national physique of our now urban
civilisation to what it was when we were for the
most part rural ; if our C 3 nation, as it undoubtedly
is, imperatively needs transforming into the A 1
type which alone can maintain our place in the sun—
we need a greatly increased supply of safe milk.
All proposals, however promising or desirable in
themselves, which would have the effect of reducing
a supply, already disastrously inadequate, are *ipso
facto* condemned.

Our national need requires us to appeal to the

modern dairyman for his help, which is our absolutely indispensable and first requirement. Can he, will he, do for us what we require ? The answer to the first question is affirmative ; what I have actually seen him doing I clearly know that he can do. Whilst we await the unquestionably desirable reform in the farm, milk from many farms, where reform may be desired but is not yet attained, pours into our great cities with its inevitable dirt and living bacilli. Such milk can be and is being cleaned by means of the centrifuge, and freed from infection by means of (genuine and not nominal) pasteurisation. But these precautions are futile if the milk is to be, as usually hitherto, contaminated in the home. Of what avail our Listerian milkmen and shaven cows at the farm (supposing that we had them) when " there's many a slip 'twixt the cup and the lip " ? We want the milk to be safe when it reaches the lip, whatever it was or was not before that crucial moment.

These things can be done efficiently and on the grand scale if the dairyman is merely prepared to give his life to his work, to train skilled workers, to spend thousands of pounds on the necessary apparatus and service. Then he asks the public for, say, an extra penny a quart—though how that can begin to suffice I cannot imagine—and promptly his fellow-countrymen live up to Carlyle's description of them and decline to pay. For a penny less per quart they prefer to buy their milk *plus* all manner of muck and microbes, ready to poison and destroy themselves and their children. Scotland spends about seven times as much on whisky as on milk, and the pitiful children of the great Scottish cities— the population of most of which is actually declining according to the figures of the last census—are the resultant commentary on this colossal and calamitous national folly.

The answer to the second question, therefore, whether the dairyman will do what he certainly can for us depends on the public. Or perhaps it depends on persons like myself who call themselves doctors, which means *teachers*, as to whether or not we can and will teach these many well-meaning people.

If I may pledge myself, at any rate, as a lover and student of national health, my pen and voice are here pledged to this essential task. What they can do shall be done. Here's out against the beery superstition of to-day and for the " pure milk of the word " of to-morrow !

As if to link up sunlight and milk, these two agents of normal nutrition and vital resistance, even more closely than we have already shown, Hess and his fellow-workers have made a series of observations which mean, in effect, that milk of perfect composition can be produced only by cows which are properly sunlit and fed on green leaves—which are themselves the product of sunlight. Evidently there is here a lesson for the nursing mother and those who care for her, as well as for all who are concerned in the production and use of milk. It may be that, in view of the new American work, we must recognise two vitamins, similar in some respects but distinct, which have hitherto been subsumed under the term vitamin A. It remains to be seen what are the relations between "vitamin A" and "vitamin A 1"; but in any case the experimental record is to the effect that when young animals are fed exclusively on the milk produced by cows fed in the shade and on a vitamin-free fodder, it does not suffice for their needs; they lose weight and die. On the other hand, similar animals fed on similar quantities of the milk of cows fed on pasture (which involves the action of sunlight both on the cows and on the green leaves they consume), grow and thrive. In the first experiments along these lines, which we are quoting, vitamin C appears to have been chiefly concerned, but doubtless the same general principle is involved in the other cases. Not vitamins alone are concerned. "Passing over minor variations," say our authors, "it is seen that the percentages of calcium and of phosphorus were significantly higher in the pasture milk, and that its citric acid content was over 50 per cent. greater."[1]

There remains one particularly interesting possibility which brings sunlight and milk as closely as possible together, and applies the findings above quoted. We can, in effect, bring over Antipodean sunlight to this country, in any quantities, treasured up for use in the form of dried milk which has been produced by cows feeding in sunlight and on pasture all the year round; and by means of the abundant

[1] "Relation of Fodder to the Antiscorbutic Potency and Salt Content of Milk," by Alfred F. Hess, N. J. Unger and G. C. Supplee (*Journal of Biological Chemistry*, December, 1920).

vitamins and salts which it contains we can make good the deficiencies inevitable in the milk produced by our own cows during the winter.

Evidently we do not yet know whether the sunlight acts in the fodder or upon the cow, or both. The Lister Institute is now investigating this important point.

CHAPTER XIV

SUNLIGHT AND CHILDHOOD: A CHAPTER
FOR MOTHERS.

WHEN "the year's at the spring," we feel something stirring in our bones; it is the light of life, the returning sun, immediate author of the fire that burns, be it sluggish or brilliant, in the bodies of all living things. In this chapter we pass from even the food of foods back to the sunlight, the source of all foods, the stimulant and tonic and healer incomparable, the rediscovery of which is the greatest medical event in many decades. The knife and the bottle have their uses, but the cult of the knife and the bottle has degraded the healing art, until there is no beautiful and subtle structure in our bodies but the surgeon itches to remove it, whilst we bestow the lovely name of spring medicine upon various chemical aperients, and forget the real spring medicine, the blessed sun, which arises with healing in its wings.

This is of the very stuff of which poetry is made, and poetry is supposed to be the antithesis of science. Before discussing the way in which we should order our lives, and our children's, under the orient sun, I propose therefore to re-state, in the coldest terms, the most recent findings of science about the sunlight and the spring.

At Columbia University and the Home for Hebrew Infants, in New York—which I revisited in December, 1922, in order to see this work at first hand—it has been found, for the first time in the history of science, that the sunlight controls the chemistry of the blood. Continuous observations, begun in 1921, have shown that, on a constant diet, the quantity of phosphorus in the blood of an infant or young child is at a minimum in March, begins to go up in April, rises until July, and then slowly but steadily descends until March again. Observations begun a little later show the same curve for the lime of the blood. It has long been known that the amount of red stuff, containing iron, in the blood increases when one lives in the mountains ; and I have always, therefore, refrained from accepting the statement that the Alpine sun-cure enriches the blood in iron, thanks to the light alone, until we had more evidence ; but it has now been proved that light, as such, apart from any mountains, adds to the iron in the blood. In the urban laboratories of New York, at no altitude, and in ordinary stagnant urban air, the action of light has been shown even to double the phosphorus content of an infant's blood in a fortnight, on an unchanged diet.

It has also been shown that, in certain instances, poisons which would be fatal in their action during the darker months of the year are resisted in the late spring and summer. A famous skin specialist, with whom I was lately discussing some proposals for the increased use of sunlight, told me, to my delight, that, when any of his juniors was proposing a new treatment for an intractable chronic skin disease—known as *lupus erythematosus*—he told them to be sure to begin the new treatment in the spring, and then they would get good results !

Lastly, it has been shown that the thyroid gland in the neck, the use of which, we know, will cure idiocy, due to lack of it, is richer in its unique iodine-containing secretion in the summer than in the winter. We thus have the definitely proved beginnings of a seasonal chemistry of the sunlight, and upon this the new medicine will be based.

Now, observe the use of calcium and phosphorus in bone building, note the annual curve of those elements in babies' blood ; and consider the discovery that, in New York—a smokeless city which only has mild cases of rickets in the light-starved slums of its lower east side—no new cases of rickets occur in summer, and the largest number of new cases begin in March. It is, as I called it years ago, before this discovery, a " disease of darkness." But, long before myself, an English doctor had found the truth, and proclaimed its lessons.

In the garden of England, at an advanced age, the holder of no honorary degrees or public distinctions, still practising his profession, lives the true victor of rickets, the man who, after the medical profession had been studying " the English disease " for centuries in vain, found the profound and simple truth about it.

In 1890, in two numbers of the *Practitioner*, having used such methods as were available to a

medical missionary on a remote station, writing to
friends and colleagues throughout the world and
collating their data, Dr. Theobald Adrian Palm
proved that the chief factor in the causation of
rickets is deprivation of sunlight. He and his work,
though published in a leading journal, under the
editorship of Sir Lauder Brunton, were absolutely
ignored. He is not mentioned in the historical
records of rickets published by the Medical Research
Council, and I found his name in America,
thanks to the thoroughness with which an
American bibliographer of the sunlight had done
his work.

Our country has suffered incalculable injury,
countless persons have died, countless more are
deformed or enfeebled to-day, because Dr. Palm's
great discovery of a generation ago was ignored,
and has yet to be applied in our children's hospitals
and in our urban lives. I place him high among
the number of those few in the nineteenth century—
the last of the ages of darkness—whom I call heralds
of the dawn, and I count it a rare privilege to pay
him public honour at long last, when the laboratory
chemists of two continents (for the American work
mentioned above has now been confirmed by our
own students) are vying with each other in the
cumulation of exact experimental records that he
was right.

I have never had the honour of meeting Dr. Palm,
but I have read his " Faith of an Evolutionist," and
can guess that if this belated publicity (for which I
take sole responsibility) be at all to his liking, the

only reason must be that he hopes for a consequent amelioration of the state of our nation's childhood. There is no space here to discuss the technical parts of his paper, but I will answer, after thirty-three years, his question of 1890. " It would be interesting to know how emigrants, from the classes in Europe which produce most rickety children, are affected by removal to climes where they enjoy more sunshine." *In Canada I have never seen a case of rickets in four successive years ; I have met many doctors who did not even know to what kind of disease the name refers.*

Doubtless the reader asks how to use sun baths, as well he may. I do not regard this question as of the first importance, for the essential things to do are to abolish our coal-smoke and our slums, to equip our houses and factories accordingly, and to live more in the open air, without the usual preposterous excess of skin covering, and thus to get our sun baths, at work and at play and in the ordinary course of our lives, whilst we are thinking of something else.

That is how people get their sun baths in North America, and it illustrates the principle of natural prevention, and also the profoundly important principle of living a healthy life and forgetting all about " health " and " treatment " and doctors. (No one can be healthy who is always consciously trying to be healthy. The mind should be turned outwards, not within.) But it is a very proper thing to think of the health of others, and there is much need for systematic use of sun baths in the treatment

doctors in other countries have treated consumption of the lungs by exposure to the mid-day sun, with the most tragic results in some cases, because the heat of the sun has killed the patients. That, if it were a cure, might be called the heat-cure, but it is utterly unlike the sun-cure in its principles and its results.

The truth is that the sun-cure is not a simple, obvious, easy method which any one can apply to anybody, as too many people suppose. More accidents yet will happen, and many disappointments, until those concerned are prepared to read the one authoritative and comprehensive volume in our language, or, at least, to learn from those who have visited the cliniques of Dr. Rollier and spent day after day in watching the true sun-cure applied. Once again, therefore, I sound a clear note of warning, and, as the person most responsible for the arrival of the sun-cure in England, I definitely repudiate responsibility for the results of ignorant or careless use of so potent and complex an agent as the sun's rays upon our bodies, each of which has its own special personal qualities, and none of which can be helped by the sun or by any other medicine or kind of treatment except in so far as it responds rightly thereto.

The rule of rules is *hasten slowly*. Using the powerful Alpine sun upon weakly patients, with bloodless, flabby, pale, light-starved skins, Dr. Rollier follows a general plan, which is to expose the feet only, for only five minutes at a time, perhaps twice or thrice the first day, and thence, gradually exposing the limbs more and longer, to exposure of the trunk, until, at the end of a fortnight, the patient may be entirely bathed in the light for three or even four hours. This I write merely to give the general idea. The times and figures do *not* apply to any particular case. Every case, even that of a well child or adult whom one wishes to benefit by the sunlight, and much more the case of a sick person, must be watched and guided by *the way in which it responds* to the light. That response is everything. Without it the light can do no more than it could for a corpse. Results to fear and be warned by are named above. No such result should ever occur ; all may quickly occur unless we are careful and intelligent.

The sun-cured person begins to turn brown. This pigmentation of the skin is very important. We do not understand it, and we are now studying it in many new and special ways. The patient who pigments deeply and quickly is the patient who quickly profits by the light and recovers. If people freckle only, they must hasten more slowly than ever. Red-haired people are often refractory in this fashion, and we must be patient with them. With time and care they will usually brown nicely and evenly, and all will go well.

The head must be protected and the eyes be shaded by a linen hat or otherwise. Sunstroke and eye-strain may easily follow neglect of these simple precautions, which have nevertheless been often neglected. As in everything else, different persons' heads and eyes vary widely in this respect. Some eyes, in the Alps, even need shaded glasses, especially in the winter, clad in brilliant snow.

Since the heat of the sun enervates, depresses, exhausts, burns, and otherwise does exactly the opposite of all we desire, we must use those hours of the day which give us the light rather than the heat. Here is new and most cogent evidence in favour of the principle of daylight saving. The early morning hours are best. At Leysin, in the summer, Dr. Rollier can use no others. In India, as a distinguished Indian physician whom I met at Leysin in 1922 pointed out to me, the sun is so hot so early that, on his return, he proposed to experiment with filters, which should arrest the terrible, dangerous heat and let through the beneficent light with healing in its wings. That, of course, is what Finsen showed and did long ago, having a stream of cold water always running between two quartz lenses, so that the quartz and the water let through the precious light and ultra-violet rays to the spot of lupus on the young cheek, whilst the heat rays were absorbed by the cool stream of water. The sun-cure is the sun*light*-cure, and the heat of the sun is a complication and enemy which we must avoid.

We cannot live without water, but this does not mean that we must drink it continuously. It is possible to have too much of a good thing. Dr. Rollier never exposes any patient to all the sunlight of the day. Three or four hours of the intense Alpine sun is a full dose. Dosage comes in here as with everything else that has ever been heard of. The mothers of over-stimulated and excited and sleepless children who have been playing nearly nude all day on the shore in July, in the sun's light and heat, should understand this proposition.

" Baths of water are good, baths of air are better, baths of light are best." That is a saying of the French students, and we know it to be true, by sheer exact proof in the research laboratories in New York and Vienna and elsewhere.

The beach is incomparable. It gives the child everything. If we use it well, we need not regret the Swiss mountains. But we must use it with intelligence. The glorious records of Dr. Rollier at Leysin, or of Sir Henry Gauvain at the Treloar Homes at Alton and Hayling Island, depend upon the use of natural means, with special and critical reference to each particular child and its particular response to the means employed. Yet again, therefore, I must say that I can only state principles.

The evident danger points are two, the head and the eyes. If we could really get our children on to the beach soon after dawn, and obtain their unique value from those early morning hours, bright and cool, which are only a rumour for most of us, there would be little need to warn parents that *the heat of the sun*, beyond a very low point, is not our friend.

But I cannot say, with any hope of being followed, " Get up really early, for the best of the day, ' so sweet, so cool and bright,' and ' fear no more the heat of the sun.' " What I must say is that a loose, light, perforated, white, soft, linen hat—or cap with a brim all round if that describes it better—is the proper headgear for children under the July sun.

It is the thing that boys wear when playing cricket, the thing the Australian and South African cricketers use, the thing worn by all at Leysin, and it is ideal for the purpose. Under it the head may be kept reasonably cool, and the brim shades the eyes and the back of the neck, which is a danger point, since there the spinal cord, as it leaves the shelter of the skull and runs down inside the backbone, comes near the surface. With this precaution, in this country, the risk of sunstroke, which is almost always, or always, heat stroke, may be entirely avoided.

Remember dosage and the " golden mean." It is possible to have too much of a good thing ; a baby may even have too much of its mother's arms.

The common sense of paddling is that the child on the beach is right in wanting to paddle, thus getting baths of water and air and light, in some degree. Sir Henry Gauvain obtains excellent results from having the children at Hayling Island, suffering from tuberculosis, go paddling and bathing in the sea. (Those who cannot walk can be carried in and dipped.)

Bathing is better than paddling, and a child can scarcely be too young to learn to swim. As ever, the response of life to what is offered it is everything. Some one has blundered, something is wrong if the child on the beach has a headache or cannot eat or cannot sleep. But if we do not blunder, we shall see for ourselves what Nature can do when her children respect and try to understand her.

Here, in order of increasing importance, are certain

tasks which, I think, in view of our new discoveries, devolve upon the women of Great Britain, because the men alone have proved quite incapable of discharging them.

1. Within reasonable limits, curtains and blinds and shutters must be drastically restricted, except for use at night. *We have enough sunlight in England, but only if we value and use it.* Do we prefer to see a good colour in our carpets or in our children's cheeks ? To some extent we must choose, but to that extent the choice cannot be in doubt. It is time to end the folly of spending time and money in the purchase of pills and capsules and liquid chemicals, rich in iron, lime and phosphorus, and dosing our children with them, in the shade, now that we have learnt how sunlight dominates the chemistry of the blood, and how, on the simplest and most inexpensive diet of natural foods, the blood will contain all the precious things it needs, given sunlight.

We must include window-glass with blinds and shutters, for it is opaque, most unfortunately, to the most powerfully vital rays that the sun sends us—the ultra-violet or " chemical " rays.

2. *We must not allow fashion to dominate our clothing, or ourselves, or our children.* We must aim at health, which is a first condition of beauty, and beauty is always fashionable, except in the eyes of fools, " by whom to be dispraised were no small praise." Short of entirely denuding our limbs, we can choose materials which allow some valuable light to pass through. I obtained in Columbia

University last year samples of an inexpensive
mercerised cotton, one black and the other white,
in the same material. Through the former, light
will not cure rickets ; through the latter it will.
These researches have only just been begun. They
tend towards more liberal and innocent ideas of
the human body and its clothing than our grand-
mothers might have approved, and away from a
kind of prudery which was a poor substitute for
nice-minded modesty. At my request, Professor
Leonard Hill has repeated, at Hampstead, the
observations of Hess, in New York, and has confirmed them. Miss M. B. Synge, a well-known
student of children's clothing,* has, upon my
suggestion, adopted certain materials, in conformity
with these results, for what she calls " sunshine
clothing," and exhibited some of the products at
our Infant Welfare Conference in London in Baby
Week, 1923.

3. Women have to make homes of life out of the
houses of brick built by men. New houses are to be
built. Women should effectively demand, through
their representatives, that in these new houses,
smokeless equipment shall be provided, as urged by
the Ministry of Health's Committee of Smoke
Abatement and ignored by the Ministry in its New
Bill for Smoke Abatement.

Also, it needs the women of the country, as trustees
of its children, to counteract the influence of the big

* See her chapter, " The Clothing of Infants," in *Mothercraft*,
published by the National League of Health, Maternity and Child
Welfare, 117, Piccadilly, W.

manufacturers who are now telling the Government that industry will be ruined unless factory chimneys are to smoke as ever. Essen, Cologne, Dusseldorf, Zurich, New York (for instance) are smokeless. If our manufacturers cannot conduct their businesses without destroying the people, they should yield to others who can. Meanwhile, by their " works " we shall know them.

I beseech my readers for their help in this public and national matter, which is part of our duty to the nation's childhood, our sacred trust. We should demand action at once lest it be said, when the smog, as I call the combination of aqueous fog and coal-smoke, returns each autumn, " The harvest is past, summer is ended, and we are not saved."

CHAPTER XV

THE SCHOOL IN THE SUN

WE were some sixty medical men and women, all in practice save myself, and mostly responsible for tuberculous patients in all parts of the world—London, Paris, Philadelphia, Madras, and so forth. We walked downhill a mile or two from Leysin, and then sat in the shade, in our foolish clothes, and watched a company of uproariously happy children at school in the sun. They were assembled, like ourselves, from all parts of the world, to live in the light of the sun and of real science, based upon Nature, and buttressed by every method and mechanism of contemporary research. These were the children of " L'Ecole au Soleil," established in 1910 by Dr. Rollier, the Prometheus-Æsculapius of Leysin, and described by him in a delightful little book of that name, a translation of which into English lies in my desk at home, awaiting the moment when some publisher will show enough interest and pluck to publish it. These children have all been persistently ill at home, in one or another of the great capitals of what we call civilisation. In the winter they get bronchitis and colds and sore throats and " glands in the neck " and anæmia, and other specimens of the diseases of darkness, and the only way to save

them, after they have swallowed vast quantities of
hypophosphites and cod liver oil, and so forth, is to
send them up here, where they flourish exceedingly.
The pen of John Ruskin is needed to describe the
school, as we saw it in action ; nor can I here show
the film which illustrates the school in summer and
in winter. But we heard the children discuss the
botany, systematic and economic, of the mushroom ;
they sang in chorus ; they recited ; they did physical
exercises ; showed us high jumping and the tug-of-
war. The intellectual part of the lesson was not a
joke or a pretence, but thoroughly solid. People
suppose such a school to be a sort of burlesque :
" as if one could only be serious in a prison," said
its inventor to me. The ages of the children were
from four to twelve. They were boys and girls.
Their only clothing was one or another variety of
loin cloth, a linen hat, and shoes. Their happy little
bodies were exposed to the sun, and their skins
were deeply pigmented by its light. No noses were
running ; I heard no cough, despite much very
active exertion ; and it was the happiest school-
class I have ever seen in my life. How highly such
happiness should be rated we can realise only if we
try to imagine what would be the condition of those
children if they were not here. Such children are
lying in the shade in hospitals all over England,
patiently suffering until they die. On their behalf
I protest against the insular inertia and scepticism
which dooms all these children to death by darkness
whilst the clinicians stand with their backs to the
light, their shadows on their patients, and pronounce

their prognosis. The hapless children do not know enough to make Diogenes' reply to Alexander.

When first I visited Leysin I was ignorant enough to suppose that I had not time to visit the school in the sun. But I made one attempt thereafter to see something of the sort. As is worth repeating, a medical friend took me to see a sanatorium for tuberculous children in the far north of England, the first of its kind in our country, and he promised me that I should see the use of the sun at home. The place is close to the east coast, in a position as hopelessly and impossibly unsuitable as could almost anywhere be found, and the sun was not shining. The schoolmistress told me that the children lived largely in the open air, " and when the sun shines, we go into that wood," she added, pointing a short distance away. The reason given was that the doctors ordered this as a precaution for the children's eyes.

It is not the business of the five practitioners from England who were at Leysin in August, 1922, to advocate a revolution in our ideas of the conditions under which children should be taught in school ; and the laws of medical ethics interfere with free expression on the part of those who might thus be regarded as attracting patients to their consulting rooms. But it is my privilege to say that what we saw that afternoon is a needed lesson for all the world, and for our country most of all. We all need to go to school in the sun.

Phosphorus is a good thing in a child's blood. So is calcium. No child nor man can live without these things ; nor bones nor teeth can be formed without them. We supply them copiously in medicinal form, therefore, and the idea is excellent. Very often we fail, however, to get the results we desire. But the Americans have shown, and our own workers are confirming them, that, without any amelioration of a thoroughly vicious and defective diet, the amount of phosphorus in the blood will be doubled after a week or two of daily exposure, lasting a few minutes only, to sunlight. Some chemical process is thus begun, some ferment, or internal secretion, or " hormone," constructed, which enables the body to take and keep and use, from the diet, what it would otherwise have to go without. And the children at the school in the sun, most inexpensively and simply fed, without any medicine or cod liver oil, flourish and grow strong and straight, and remain so, doubtless because these mysterious and as yet unexamined vital processes are set going in their bodies by the prime source of all life and health.

It was very impressive to me to hear from the clinicians at Leysin during that week in August, 1922, how entirely unprecedented in their experience were the results they saw. Being no clinician myself, and not being acquainted at first hand with the results to-day obtained otherwise than by sunlight, I was, of course, very fortunate to hear such expressions from those who are professionally engaged in the treatment of tuberculosis in various parts of the world.

But for me, and for all but an unfortunate minority of my present readers, the significance of helio-

therapy is in what it teaches us for *heliohygiene*.
The clinic in the sun leads us to the school in the sun.
Some people are indignant that I should reiterate
the praises of a foreign doctor, to whom our patients
may desire to go. They fail to see the point. As I
have repeatedly written and said in public, and to
Dr. Rollier himself, my object is not to add to the
number of his patients, but to rob him of all patients
and leave him with nothing to do but stroll round
one after another of his thirty-seven clinics, dictating
the memoirs which the empty beds call to his mind.
The real meaning of Leysin is that the continued
existence of tuberculosis (and *à fortiori*, of rickets)
is a scandal and a disgrace to our civilisation.
These diseases should be known to students of
medical history, and to them alone. As scurvy is a
" deficiency disease," due to lack of vitamin C, and
as we end scurvy on our ships or during Polar
expeditions by supplies of lime or lemon juice, and
end scurvy in our babies by a daily teaspoonful of
orange juice, so tuberculosis and rickets should be
looked upon as deficiency diseases also, the lacking
agent of health in these instances being sunlight.

To Sir James Dewar, our veteran chemist, now
dead, I owe, in conversation which he allowed me
to quote, and in references to his lectures at the
Royal Institution decades ago, some valuable data
regarding the pioneers who showed the distinction
between the light of the sun and the heat of the sun.
Elsewhere * I have discussed this question, and

* See a detailed paper in *The World's Health*, the journal of the
League of Red Cross Societies, September, 1922.

noted the remoteness of the date at which our own Priestley and others showed that, for instance, it is not the heat but the light of the sun by which plants live and make their chlorophyll and create the substances upon which all animals, including ourselves, depend for their lives. Those persons who cannot distinguish between light and heat should leave this subject alone ; they have already delayed most deplorably the coming day when the prevention and cure of pulmonary tuberculosis will be achieved by sunlight. In all times and places, where men have reason enough to serve them like the instinct of the animals in our own Zoological Gardens, or elsewhere, the sunlight can save. The early morning sunlight rejoices the chamois, as Dr. Rollier has remarked to me, but during the heat of mid-day the wise creature rests in the shade. Light stimulates, heat depresses.

Our appallingly malurbanised country had been wiser if it had remembered that not at the end but in the beginning, " God said, ' Let there be light.' "

Our object with children in the summer ought to be to keep them *cool and bright*. If we do so, and do not poison them with dirty food, there should and will be *no summer ailments*.

This is easily written but not easily done. Evidently, however, it reinforces, *inter alia*, our age-long beliefs as to the value of the early morning hours ; it strongly supports the principle of " daylight saving " ; and it furnishes new and exact scientific evidence, derived from the clinical phenomena of tuberculosis, from experimental hæmatology, and from the new experimental osteology of

recent years, for the ancient truth of experience,
which we may render anew—

> Fear the heat and love the light,
> Keep your children cool and bright :
> Early to bed and early to rise,
> Makes a child healthy, happy and wise.

CHAPTER XVI

SMOKE AND THE WORKERS, DOMESTIC AND INDUSTRIAL

I FIRST had my attention drawn to the public health aspect of domestic service when a medical student in Edinburgh a quarter of a century ago. In a volume published in 1907, I wrote as follows :—

The life, as regulated by the ordinary mistress, is a poor one ; and such a mistress is nowadays experiencing much difficulty in finding good servants or in keeping them when found. But it is a significant fact that, though similar means of selection be employed in different cases, one mistress will constantly have occasion to worry about her servants, whilst another comes across "treasures," and is able to retain them.

Doctors know how high is the proportion of illness among domestic servants, how liable they are to bloodlessness and varicose veins, flat feet, consumption and heart weakness. They fill the general hospitals, they furnish a large proportion of their patients to doctors in poor practice, and from their scanty earnings they combine to swell the enormous incomes of the owners of patent medicines. Probably a majority of all mistresses attempt to exact from their female servants an amount of work of which the average female organism is incapable, meanwhile allowing an amount of time " out " that is quite inadequate for recuperation—the more so because, being scanty, and the working time being so dull, it is usually spent in places of amusement as abominably ventilated as nearly all our public resorts are. Thus the sympathy of the doctor is with the servant rather than the mistress.

Sixteen years after, and having since paid four prolonged visits to North America, I adhere with renewed emphasis to that statement. It need only be added that the rising standard of industrial

152

hygiene since those words were written makes more conspicuous the signal lack of improvement on any large scale in domestic hygiene "below stairs"; and that the poor conditions and consequent poor health of the girls from whom the birth rate of the future, if any, is most recruited tend seriously to injure the eugenic prospect, which is in any case poor enough.

Having made my point about the public health aspect of the question, hitherto ignored, let me indicate one conspicuous means of improvement— not that there are no others, but that it will here suffice as a leading illustration of my contention.

It is doubtless true that some servants are opposed to labour-saving appliances—such as vacuum cleaners—which require to be operated by them; but, on the other hand, there can be no doubt amongst those who have enquired into the subject that the great majority of servants welcome such labour-saving devices as gas cooking stoves, gas fires and water heaters, electric radiators and oil stoves, which obviously diminish the dirty drudgery associated with the use of crude coal for cooking, heating water for baths and warming rooms.

The coal range with its soot-laden flues; the back-breaking coal scuttle to be filled in the basement cellar and carried to the upper floors; the grate full of ashes to be cleaned up in the chill hours of early morning; the chimney that will not pull, and the fire that will not draw—have they not played the leading part in creating the smutty-faced, grimy-handed, dirty-aproned drudge—the pathetic little "slavey"—who has become, on the stage and in the comic papers, the standing joke that has gone far to make domestic service unpopular and unattractive ?

That is true beyond question ; and it is further true that the same barbarous, inefficient and wasteful way of utilising our dwindling coal resources which creates soot, dust and grit within our homes, defiles likewise the atmosphere without, darkens our skies, cuts off the sun from our city streets and, making our dismal basements more dismal and depressing, and our small-windowed servants' bedrooms still darker and more unattractive, reduces the vitality and lowers the spirits of their occupants. Would it not, therefore, be within the province of any inquirers to suggest to the Government that measures making for an abatement of the smoke nuisance would at the same time help in the solution of the domestic servant problem ?

Unnecessary work is a waste ; unnecessarily dirty and objectionable work is a stupidity ; work that is both unnecessary and objectionable, and is caused by that which is directly detrimental to the public health, is a crime. The kitchen range is beyond the stage of a joke, and ought to be prohibited (if gas is regarded as too costly for water heating and warming the kitchen, a coke stove fills the bill perfectly), while a soft-coal fire should be made an offence against the public health. It would then be less difficult to get and keep a good servant. It might be added that it would also be less difficult and trying to be without one.

The foregoing is not merely theoretic.

Since the war I have regained possession of my own house in Hampstead, a semi-basement house nearly a hundred years old. In view of my researches into the correlative questions of sunlight and coal-smoke during several past years, I have installed a coke stove for heating water, which serves abundantly for three baths, all in constant use, as well as the other usual purposes of hot water. Gas for heating and electricity for lighting make the house smokeless. The domestic staff, for whom the third bath was recently installed—a second bath is provided for the servant in any good class American apartment—are respected friends of the household, and enjoy its standard of domestic hygiene. Dirt, backache, domestic hill climbing, heart strain, and the irritability of fatigue are reduced to a minimum, and at least in this instance the servant problem is solved.

In the foregoing, originally submitted as evidence to the Domestic Service Inquiry of the Ministry of Labour, in Great Britain, 1923, I showed the importance of smokeless domestic equipment in the interests of the health of the young girls who form the majority of domestic servants. I venture to attach much importance to the case there stated for smokeless housing, in order to raise the standard of domestic hygiene, especially for the domestic servant, as the standard of industrial hygiene has been raised in recent years. But I may here add that we should recognise the immense advantage to factory workers of abolishing all the heavy and dirty work associated with the combustion of coal, which is just as much detrimental to the interest of labour in factories and workshops as it is to labour in the great industry of domestic service. It has been clearly proved, in many countries, that gas can frequently take the place of coal for manufacturing processes with many advantages from the point of view of industrial profit, *e.g.*, saving of chimneys, coal storage, cartage and handling of coal and ashes, whilst the health and happiness of the workers and of their families must gain greatly.

Nothing like our deadly industrial chimneys now remains on earth. Three years ago I visited Pittsburg on three occasions in the course of this inquiry, and found that even that notorious city, once known as " hell with the lid off," had abolished 85 per cent. of its smoke. But, of course, it cannot control the smoke produced by chimneys just outside its own jurisdiction, and this is the argument for large administrative areas in this connection, and against the omission of any such provision in the Bill introduced into Parliament lately, and against the recent deplorable decision of the London County Council in declaring that this is a matter for the individual boroughs to control, which is exactly what, by the nature of the problem, it is not.

Forty-eight years have passed since any legislation on this subject, and even the clauses in the great Public Health Act of 1875 were futile, for they apply only to " black smoke." In New York and in Pittsburg my hosts laughed aloud on hearing of this farce, whereby the prosecuted manufacturer need only call a witness to say that he saw a tinge of grey or brown or any other fancy colour in the smoke, and the prosecution falls to the ground. In view of the recent discoveries about sunlight, that one word must have cost scores of thousands of lives since 1875.

The Ministry of Health appointed a committee to study the subject, and it reported unanimously, in a very moderate fashion, asking for legislation in such matters as the removal of the word " black," and the enlargement of the areas responsible, for otherwise a good area is at the mercy of its stupid neighbour's smoke, and the inspector who indicts a nuisance may be at the mercy of the manufacturer, who sits on the local council and helps to appoint the inspector. I was able to submit American evidence on both these points to the Committee. Some time ago a deputation went to Sir Alfred Mond, and we were led to hope that the Government would really do something.

But recently a deputation representing the Federation of British Industries told the Ministry of Health that no legislation should be promoted against the industrial chimney, for otherwise our industries would be ruined. They said that they did not know how to conduct their industries without the production of smoke. This I can well believe. For the most part these men inherit industries from the nineteenth century, and under their direction we are steadily losing the industrial eminence of that age. Any statement of theirs as to not knowing anything meets with my immediate acceptance.

Subsequently a deputation representing all the leading voluntary health societies of the country went to the Ministry, but I regret to say that, in Lord Onslow's courteous reply, it was evident that he had been influenced by the manufacturers. Nothing must be done to injure industry at this time, he said, with which, of course, we all agree. A Bill is now before Parliament, under which the manufacturers will be asked to reduce their smoke " as far as practicable," and the thing will be as futile as the Act of 1875. Here I warn the nation against acceptance of this cowardly and farcical measure, which ignores nearly all the essential recommendations of Lord Newton's Committee, and has evidently been drafted under fear of the lazy and incompetent and selfish manufacturers who have so long been content to destroy us.

Lord Newton and Mr. E. D. Simon, lately Lord Mayor of Manchester, went to Germany on behalf of the Committee on Smoke Abatement. They reported that Cologne and Düsseldorf and Essen were absolutely smokeless. The statement that Sheffield must make smoke or it cannot make the steel which defends us against our enemies is answered by the simple fact that Essen makes everything that Sheffield makes except the smoke. Our investigators also noted that the German manufacturers live inside their cities, whereas ours naturally live well outside the deadly filth which they produce, and in which their workers and their children have to live and die.

Amongst devices found eminently successful in

Pittsburg, I was told there, is the use of powdered coal, and of the automatic stoker. The Germans largely use gas. In Pittsburg the manufacturers talked just as ours do now, but the people were tired of being smoked to death and insisted, and now the manufacturers make more money than ever, thanks to economy of fuel and increased industrial health.

For myself, I have studied and agitated on this subject for twenty years, but I despair of any action unless the people themselves, those who cannot live in country houses and spend the winter on the Riviera, will awake and act.

During the coal strike in Britain in 1921 people were astonished at the amelioration and even the beauty of our cities. I missed this observation, being in America, but every one remarked upon it when I returned. My friend, Mr. T. W. Littleton Hay, has reminded me how the smokeless early-morning aspect of London from Westminster Bridge moved Wordsworth on September 3rd, 1803. The lovely lines may be quoted here to show our citizens how the modern Babylon might look if her citizens would abolish the smoke of her burning and restore to her the light of day :—

> " Earth has not anything to show more fair :
> Dull would he be of soul who could pass by
> A sight so touching in its majesty :
> The city now doth like a garment wear
> The beauty of the morning ; silent, bare,
> Ships, towers, domes, theatres and temples lie
> Open unto the fields, and to the sky,
> All bright and glittering in the smokeless air.
> Never did sun more beautifully steep
> In his first splendour,-valley, rock, or hill."

Note.—The student will obtain much valuable information from the following :—

Coal Smoke Abatement Society (Secretary, Lawrence Chubb, 25, Victoria Street, S.W. 1).

Coal Smoke Abatement League (Hon. Sec., John W Graham, M.A., Dalton Hall, Manchester).

These two organisations do not overlap, but co-ordinate. The former deals with London, and the latter with the industrial North.

Advisory Committee on Atmospheric Pollution (Dr. J. S. Owens, 47, Victoria Street, S.W. 1).

Committee on Smoke and Noxious Vapours Abatement. Final Report, 1922. H.M. Stationery Office, Kingsway, W.C. (6*d.* net.)

CHAPTER XVII

MORE LIGHT

BELIEF in the value of the sun is, of course, very ancient. It appears to have been assumed partly that the sun was destructive to *noxious* things—the word " noxious " being associated with *nox*, the night—and also that the light was absorbed by the body and in some way used. This assumption, however, was never examined. Modern helio-therapy may be said to date from the discovery that light is bactericidal. In a valuable address [1] delivered in 1902, Sir James Crichton-Browne discusses the matter and shows how this led on to the work of Finsen. The antiseptic action of light was thought to be sufficient to account for such results as were obtained, and since it was asserted that this action depended generally upon the ultra-violet rays, various efforts were made to improve upon the light of common day by means of artificial light richer than sunlight in those rays. At the London Hospital, Lord Knutsford tells me, they early had to abandon the use of sunlight in the Finsen treatment of lupus, and from that moment onwards the artificial has always taken precedence in interest and attention over the natural. But now the whole question is before us again in a new aspect,

[1] " Light and Sanitation " : Sherratt and Hughes, Manchester.

where the bactericidal potency of light is in the background.

Gauvain and all other observers are in agreement with the proposition of Rollier himself, that the patients who do not pigment do not respond to the treatment, and the conclusion would be that the pigmentation is protective against the ultra-violet rays, which on a former theory were supposed to contain the therapeutic virtues of light.

But this is by no means clear to me. While it may be the case that the ultra-violet rays, in the absence of pigment, do harm, we have no evidence to show that, even in its absence, they can penetrate to any but a very short distance within the tissues. An alternative explanation of the clinical facts is that pigmentation is part of the power of response to light, and the absence of pigmentation indicates a failure of that power. Some choice between these two theories might be made if we were to employ artificial screens, whether made of melanin, or otherwise, as substitutes for natural pigmentation in those patients who remain obstinately blonde-skinned and who are not benefited by the light. If such patients respond when artificially protected, or if they do not, we shall choose our theory accordingly.[1]

---

[1] Why does painting the unaccustomed skin with picric acid prevent blistering by the sun ? Is it the yellow pigment, or the antiseptic action of the acid ? This is merely one of a hundred interesting questions which we may ask. The provisional answer to it, Sir William Bayliss tells me, is that the yellow pigment absorbs the ultra-violet rays, and prevents them from reaching that particular layer of the skin where they produce the blister. " But," he adds, " the whole question is an interesting one, opening up the problem

It has been suggested by Rollier that the pigment transforms ultra-violet rays into red rays, and experiments have been quoted to the effect that such red rays can penetrate right through the body. It is further asserted that they also are bactericidal. Here, then, is a theory which would suffice to explain the results of heliotherapy in tuberculosis ; but is it true ? I am doubtful of every stage in the argument. Is the evidence good ? Who has confirmed the alleged results which are involved in this theory ? Does it consort with what modern physicists know ? The answers to these questions ought to be definite, but no one can answer them. If we were dealing with any of a hundred drugs, a voluminous literature would be available and practically every statement would have been tested and controlled in many and various ways. On this matter of the action of light no such body of evidence is available. The work has never been done. That which has been done is not confirmed, and we may be permitted to doubt whether really competent observers have ever approached certain parts of the subject.

Very striking evidence is contained in a paper [1] by Dr. Carl Sonne, of the Finsen Medical Light Institute at Copenhagen. In his view the principal action of light upon the body is due to its absorption by the blood, which is accordingly warmed. The rays above and below the visible octave of light are absorbed very little indeed ; while that very octave

as to where the rays act. Our Light Committee has been considering the matter to some extent."

[1] "Acta Medica Scandinavica," vol. liv., fasc. iv., Stockholm, 1921 : P. A. Norstedt & Sons.

to which the cornea is transparent and the retina sensitive is the octave to which the skin also is transparent—at least, in considerable degree—and sensitive. Again, of course, we need confirmation of these results, but assuming their accuracy we may well regard them with extreme interest.

In passing, we note for an instant the common embryological origin of the ocular and cutaneous tissues, which agree in their selective capacity towards a particular series of radiations. Indeed, we find ourselves bound to regard the skin as much more like the eye than we have hitherto supposed, and as capable of functioning in a fashion which, within limits, puts the entire digestive apparatus and the processes of oxidation necessary for the maintenance of the body temperature, literally in the shade. What an extraordinary contrast between the whole business of seeking, choosing, masticating, swallowing, digesting the fuel foods, respiring, combining oxygen with the carbon compounds, glucose or fat, or what not, and thus keeping the body warm —to say nothing of the formation of the long series of ferments necessary for all these processes ; and, on the other hand, the direct warming of the blood by exposure of the skin to the light !

I begin to ask myself whether we are right in our customary view that the denudation of the human skin is a loss for which clothes serve to compensate. It may be that we are greatly advantaged above the typical hairy mammal by the very fact that our skin is nude and therefore capable of serving us as its skin cannot serve it. True, we do not avail

ourselves of this advantage—if advantage it be—
except in a very small degree on exceptional occasions, or when our long deprivation of light, exposure
to infection, much surgery followed by secondary
infections, drugs, and so forth, have all but killed
us, and we strip, are sunlit and healed. According
to Sonne, the reaction of the human skin to light is
unique, and uniquely favourable. He has always
failed to cure tuberculosis in rabbits and guinea-pigs
by light, because they invariably show pyrexia under
its influence, as human beings, properly treated, do
not.

The apparently unfortunate restriction to the eye
alone of any capacity to respond to, and live by,
light impressed Milton, who puts these words into
the mouth of the blinded Samson Agonistes :—

" Since light so necessary is to life,
  And almost life itself, if it be true
  That light is in the Soul,
  She all in every part ; Why was the sight
  To such a tender ball as the eye confined
  So obvious and so easy to be quenched ?
  And not, as feeling, through all parts diffused,
  That she might look at will through every pore ? "

To-day we may reply that the capacity to respond
to and live by light is not " to the eye confined," but
" through all parts diffused." And organic evolution,
with its story of primitive, light-sensitive, cutaneous
pigment spots, foreshadowing the eye, shows us
how we underrated the possibilities of a well-lit skin.

According to an observation of Fabre, a student
of the highest reputation for accuracy, there would
appear to be at least one definite instance of the

absorption of sunlight and the conversion of its energy, not into heat, as in Sonne's experiments, which we can readily accept, but into some form in which it can be used by the muscles :—

" For seven months, without any material nourishment, they (the young of the spider called *Lycosa*) expend strength in moving. To wind up the mechanism of their muscles, they recruit themselves directly with heat and light. During the time when she was dragging the bag of eggs behind her the mother, at the best moments of the day, came and held up her pill to the sun. With her two hind legs she lifted it out of the ground into the full light ; slowly she turned it and re-turned it, so that every side might receive its share of the vivifying rays. Well, this bath of life, which awakened the germs, is now prolonged to keep the tender babes active.

" Daily, if the sky be clear, the *Lycosa*, carrying her young, comes up from the burrow, leans on the kerb, and spends hours basking in the sun. Here, on their mother's back, the youngsters stretch their limbs delightedly, saturate themselves with heat, take in reserves of motor-power, and absorb energy.

" They are motionless ; but, if I only blow upon them, they stampede as nimbly as if a hurricane were passing. Hurriedly they disperse ; hurriedly they reassemble ; a proof that, without material nourishment, the little animal machine is always at full pressure, ready to work. When the shade comes, mother and sons go down again, surfeited with solar emanations. The feast of energy at the Sun Tavern is finished for the day. It is repeated in the same way daily, if the weather be mild, until the hour of emancipation comes, followed by the first mouthfuls of solid food." [1]

Are there other instances of this ? And is this what it appears, or may there be enough oxidisable material in the young *Lycosa* to account for its movements (and other vital processes) in the absence of any material food ? What is its exact pigmentary condition ? There are simple living forms, combining

[1] " The Life of the Spider," by J. H. Fabre, translated by A. Teixeira de Mattos (Hodder & Stoughton), pp. 135–137.

some of the characteristics of animals and plants, which possess and use chlorophyll. Is it necessary to suppose that none of the higher animals can dissociate carbon dioxide in the presence of light and by means of some pigment or other ? Surely the young *Lycosa* must be studied from this point of view. Animal photo-synthesis may exist, if we look closely enough for it.

Let us take it, then, provisionally, that sunlight can be absorbed by the blood—a fine physiological discovery. But we are concerned to explain certain clinical facts. Really, does this old-new explanation suffice ? If it is merely a matter of warming the blood, could not that be done with hot baths ? Indeed, should we not expect to get good results by keeping our patients in warm rooms where the loss of heat from the body is retarded—a process thermally equivalent to warming the blood ?

Such warm rooms were used in the treatment of tuberculosis in the old days, with what appalling results we all know. Again, should any one say, as Sonne does, and Hill credits the explanation, that this *warming* of the blood by the light accounts for its therapeutics, what in the world are we to say of Gauvain when his tuberculous children are carried in nets into the cold sea at Hayling Island, with the necessary result of markedly *cooling* their blood ? Gauvain attributes great virtue to this process, which is of course not possible at Leysin, and Hill has quoted it, and he and his fellow-workers are delightedly observing the great increase in bodily combustion which follows it.

An extremely interested and disinterested observer, like myself, may be excused for asking at this point whether it is really the case that tuberculosis can be cured alike by warming the blood with sunlight or cooling it with sea water. My own view is that we scarcely know anything about the subject at all. I doubt whether we are any nearer the truth than the clinicians of the past who attributed the virtues of digitalis to a sedative action because they found that it slowed the pulse, or those others who used alcohol as a stimulant when, as we know, its essential action is narcotic—to paralyse inhibition, thereby simulating stimulation.

In my category of the diseases of darkness, I have, of course, included our typical urban anæmia. The relation of light to the formation of chlorophyll in the green plant is well known. According to a paper [1] published by Delépine thirty years ago, some " mother-substance " is formed in the cells of the skin, under the influence of light, and is the antecedent not only of the pigment of the skin, but also of the pigment of the blood. This, if true, is a very direct explanation of the simultaneous pigmentation and increase of hæmoglobin under heliotherapy. But is it true ? Surely we should know.

In passing from this aspect of pigmentation I note that albinos are generally regarded as lacking in resistance ; and also that the American negro is very subject to tuberculosis. Again, we need "more light."

[1] *Journal of Physiology*, vol. xii., 1891, p. 27.

" The sun is the best masseur," said Rollier to me, when I asked how the tone of the muscles of his patients is maintained, without exercise, massage or faradism. Beyond question the muscular condition of his patients is astonishing. At the Treloar Hospital I saw and felt the same thing. The explanation offered me by Rollier was that the blood, on its way to the skin, where it circulates so freely under heliotherapy, passes through the muscles and thus maintains their condition. I do not believe this explanation to be consonant at all with our physiological knowledge. Surely it is not the sun at all, but the cold air that stimulates the muscles, maintaining their tone and, by their metabolism, maintaining the temperature of the body. If this be, as I suppose, the true explanation, it consorts with Rollier's preference for the early morning hours for insolation, and with his experience that hot summer afternoons are quite unsuitable. In other words, the real merit of the " *climat d'altitude*," to which he attaches so much importance, may lie, not only, as we have been led to suppose, in its abundance of ultra-violet rays, but in its cold ; and the virtue of sea bathing, as practised by Gauvain at Hayling Island, may be not at all as an alternative to, substitute for, or equivalent of, the sun of Leysin, but as equivalent to the cold Alpine air. Clearly to think and rightly to interpret in this matter is vital for practice, let us remember, no less than for accurate physiological conclusions.

Two of the distinguished men already named above, who are working at this subject, have spoken

and written of the increased heat production of
sea-bathed children as very valuable. Clearly, if
the body is to lose much heat, by being immersed
in cold water, much heat must be made within it,
or the body temperature will fall, and if the workers
of the Medical Research Council, now studying
balneotherapy at Hayling Island, find tissue-com-
bustion much increased, as they do, we could expect
no other. But this is by no means proof of the
value of water-baths, as against heliotherapy, or
anything else. It is merely an obvious and everyday
instance of adaptation to environment on the part
of a warm-blooded animal. Yet we are asked to
believe that this directly bears upon the cure of
tuberculosis. On the contrary, no causal *nexus*
whatever has been shown or even suggested between
the compensatory combustion following cooling of
the blood and the cure of tuberculosis. In the
absence of any conjecture as to such a causal relation
between the two processes, I am not inclined to
regard cold sea bathing as in any sense a substitute
for or equivalent of heliotherapy. Indeed, how can
any one do so ?

We all speak with contempt to-day of the old
" shot-gun " prescription whereby, as Voltaire said,
the physician poured a motley assemblage of " drugs
of which he knew little into a body of which he knew
less." If and when such a prescription did good, the
question remained as to the constituent or consti-
tuents, or combination thereof, in which the virtue
resided. A similar difficulty arises in a new form
now, when we are trying to cure by more natural

and rational means. Two clinicians, such as Rollier
and Gauvain, for instance, obtain similar results,
each by a certain combination of means—the modern
rational equivalent of the " shot-gun " prescription
of yore. Each clinician, as a good follower of
Hippocrates, must use all the means he believes likely
to help his patients. They are patients, not experimental material. Each, obtaining good results,
thinks, and reasonably may, that his particular
combination of means is *the* formula for success.
We need scientific inquiry so that we may learn
exactly what ingredients, so to say, of Rollier's
prescription are really effective and what superfluous.
It is high time, surely, as my discussion above of
the procedures of respectively warming and cooling
the blood may indicate. As for ultra-violet rays, in
the latest view, I can readily foresee some one using
glass or other means whereby they can be completely
obstructed from his patients, and obtaining results,
perhaps, comparable to Rollier's without any of the
very rays to which he attaches, or has until recently
attached, such high importance. The whole matter
is in the crudely empirical pre-scientific stage of
pharmaceutical therapeutics before pharmacology.

Again, as regards air and light, it needs to be
shown that the light has special efficacy. If not,
the bearing of this work on, for instance, the records
and prospects of our open-air sanatoria for tuberculosis in this country becomes remote and dubious.
But Rollier and his fellow-workers are positive and
produce unlimited evidence ; and the recent results
obtained in stale, urban air in New York, Copenhagen

and London by the carbon arc lamp are decisive.
At Leysin the sun is often obscured, perhaps for days
at a time. The spontaneous elimination of a piece
of dead bone under the influence of insolation may
be observed to undergo arrest when the clouds
interfere with the actual sun-cure ; the sequestrum
may begin to retrace its course ; and when the sun
returns, the excretory and healing process is resumed.
That is the evidence ; and surely the fact depends
on more than either the warming of the blood or
the bactericidal action of the light. There is some
kind of vital reaction involved. And, if the reader
should think that phrase too mystical, let him be
reminded that the minutest trace of such an
anæsthetic as chloroform completely arrests the
photo-synthesis effected by chlorophyll in the
presence of sunlight. We need " more light."

Assuredly pure air and sunlight will be vindicated,
and the more so the more we inquire. My case
against the coal smoke of our cities will be acknow-
ledged to be overwhelming by every one, I predict,
when the work for which I now ask is done.

Light and heat are so closely associated in our
ordinary experience that we find it hard to couple
" light and cold " as I have persistently sought to
do in discussing this subject ; nor is the commoner
coupling of ideas less likely to prevail if it be indeed
true that the chief virtue of light is to be transformed into heat in the blood. But let us remember
the cold, sunny Canadian winter ; and the laboratory
work of Hill ; and the nude, sunlit children in the
cold air of Leysin, or the cold water off Hayling

Island ; and we shall begin to be able to think in terms of the combination of light and cold. Sonne's experiments in Copenhagen show, we have noted, that the skin is affected very differently by heat rays and light rays, the former burning and blistering the surface, while the latter are usefully absorbed. (Recent work on soft and hard Röntgen rays suggests a close parallel.) It follows that we must distinguish between light and heat at every moment in our study of this subject. Certainly we have confused sun stroke proper with heat stroke for decades enough, and there is no excuse now for failing to distinguish between the different parts of the ethereal gamut (if that be what it is) when we learn how profoundly different are the physiological reactions to them.

The failure so to distinguish was one of the errors which vitiated the most misleading and unfortunate article contributed by a fine worker, the late Professor Benjamin Moore, F.R.S., to *The Times*.[1] Though Sonne's work had already been published, and though Hill and others, including myself, have been trying to distinguish between heat and light for a long time past, in their physiological and clinical relations, Moore asked, of " summer time," " Is this greater exposure to heat and light beneficial to our health, or the reverse ? " The question, as I pointed out [2] in the ensuing correspondence, is illegitimate. It confounds two things, markedly and demonstrably

---

[1] " Summer Time and Health : Can we Have too much Sunshine ? " October 3rd, 1921.
[2] *Times*, October 5th.

different in their action upon us. Moore also called sunlight " lethal," and said that living things must protect themselves against it, and " that is why the leaves are green." Here, verily, Professor Moore forgot himself. We had to rub our eyes and remind ourselves that a writer of the same name and history was one of the foremost living students of the fundamental function of chlorophyll upon which, thanks to sunlight, the whole living world depends ! In the presence of a proper body of knowledge on this subject, such as we have on many others, vastly more complex and less important, it would have been impossible for so distinguished a student to expose himself to such overwhelming destructive criticism, and to injure the causes of biology, hygiene and medicine as he did. No one who had seen Leysin or Alton, or opened " La Cure de Soleil," or seen the children of sunny Canada, could have used such language of the light of day. Again I say, we need " more light."

In Sonne's view, all our ideas hitherto are wrong. The action of light is specific beyond question. (What a pity that we talk about " open-air " treatment, and forget the light.) But it is not chemical, but calorific. To my question mooted above—If calorific, why do not other measures for warming the blood act as well ?—the reply of Sonne is that no other measures warm the blood as the " universal light bath " does. The ultra-violet he dismisses. The red and yellow rays, in the energy of which sunlight is incomparably superior to all artificial luminants, do the work. Properly used, they warm the blood without inducing general pyrexia, with its evil consequences. Reading his paper I feel strongly supported in my contention for the value of the combination of *light* and *cold*, and in my criticism of Moore's question as illegitimate. Sonne concludes :—

" The current view that the therapeutic effect of the universal light bath should be essentially due to the ultra-violet (or the so-called chemically active) rays has not been sufficiently warranted in spite of assiduous research and numerous experiments.

" Based on a series of various facts concerning the specific absorption relations of the light rays (visible heat rays) during radiation to the human skin, the following theory is advanced : *the curative effect of the universal light bath is due to the capacity of the luminous rays, during the light bath, to heat a very essential portion of the aggregate blood volume of the organism to a temperature possibly exceeding the highest fever temperature ever measured without causing the body temperature to rise in any appreciable degree.* [Italics in original.]

" According to which the light-bath will be able to produce the inciting effect of fever upon, for instance, the oxidation and the formation of anti-bodies without producing the usual harmful effects of fever upon the organism."

Clearly these findings must be examined further.[1] Meanwhile we must not forget, if we should seem to be about to discard the ultra-violet rays, that Hess has proved their value in the mercury vapour quartz lamp, and that they are certainly bactericidal —an action of which Sonne himself says that " in point of hygienics [it] is of the highest importance." The infamous " smogs " which we endure in London and our other cities involve the loss of the cleansing virtues of sunlight and the survival of unthinkable

[1] Sir William Bayliss tells me that this is now being done under the auspices of his committee.

numbers of tubercle bacilli, in our homes and streets and elsewhere, which would otherwise have been killed. While we pursue the new clinical clue of Sonne, let us not forget the certain facts of the hygiene of sunlight.

In any case, it is, I believe, clear that the elucidation of the action of sunlight is the next great task for the medical sciences, and that the restoration of sunlight to our cities is the next great task for hygiene in this country. We need the physicist, the chemist, the biochemist, the physiologist, the clinician and the sanitarian for these tasks, and the outcome of their labours will certainly be " MORE LIGHT."